Essential Oils Collection:

73 Natural, Non-Toxic Homemade Recipes for Hair Care and

Best Organic Lotions

Table of content:

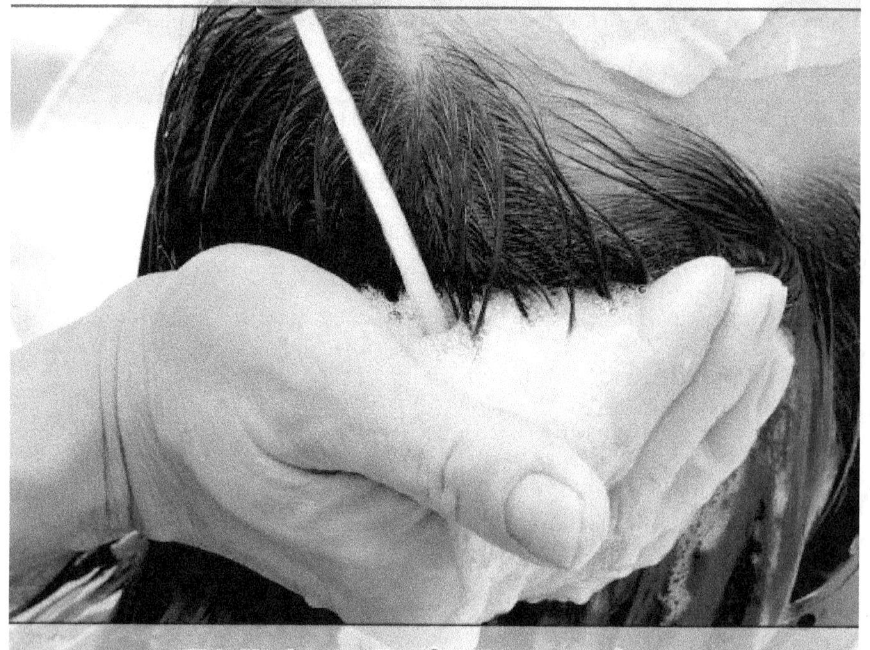

Homemade
Hair Care

34 Natural Toxic-Free Recipes
With Essential Oils For Your Hair

Donna Nolan

Homemade Hair Care:

34 Natural Toxic-Free Recipes with Essential Oils for Your Hair

Introduction: You're tired of the chemicals.

You've tried just about every hair product out there to make your hair look and feel healthy. The problem is the more you paid, the more chemicals were in the products and the more you had to purchase to cleanse your hair of the residue. You started looking online for a natural alternative, but your head spun with all the recipes, advice, and ingredients, not knowing which was actually good for your hair and which ones you needed to avoid. This book will provide, not only the answers you're looking for, but the breakdown of all the ingredients and recipes to start making your own at home. From what you need to how to make it, we will give you all you need to take charge of your own scalp and hair health.

Chapter 1 - Your Scalp and Hair

You scratch it when it itches. You scratch it when you brush it, and you pull it when you style your hair. It's your scalp, and it needs as much attention as your hair. If you scalp is dry or unhealthy, it reflects in your hair, making it either dull and dry, or oily.

Dandruff

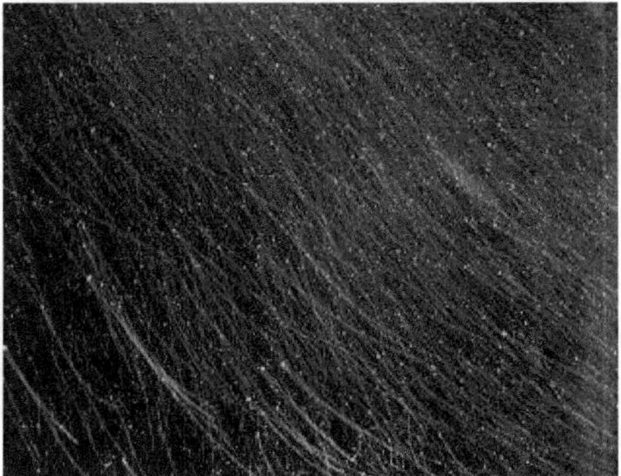

This is the flaking of your scalp when its too dry to retain the natural sebum the sabaceous glands produce. These flakes can be small, only being seen when you scratch your scalp, or large enough to be noticed by anyone who looks.

How your hair gets damaged

Your hair takes a ton of abuse. With every curling or straightening iron and blow drying session, your hair can sustain damage. You can dry out your hair when you wash it too often, over style it, and even bleach and dye your hair. Doing any of these things can leave your hair dry, stringy, brittle, and very susceptible to breaking and split ends.

When you shampoo and condition your hair, it's clean, a little too clean in some instances, making your scalp work overtime to make the sebum, or natural oil, to keep itself moisturized. This can lead to hair looking oily just 24 hours after you have washed it. There is a way to reset the balance to your scalp. It's called the:

No Shampoo Method

You only need the following ingredients to get started:
Baking soda
Water
Unfiltered Apple Cider Vinegar
Empty shampoo bottle
Two-cup measuring cup

• In a standard size bottle of water, add two tsp of baking soda and shake until it mixes into the water.

• Put a little on your palm. If it's a little slippery, than it's perfect. If not, add a little more into the water.

• In your measuring cup, add two tablespoons of apple cider vinegar.

• Fill the rest with water.

In the shower:

• Wet your hair
• Work with baking soda solution into your hair.
• Use the vinegar solution to rinse and leave it in. This will restore the pH or your scalp.

Essential Oil

It will take up to seven weeks for your hair to reset, using the technique above once a week until you don't need to use it any longer. You can add essential oils to the vinegar. Here are a couple than can help balance the scalp:

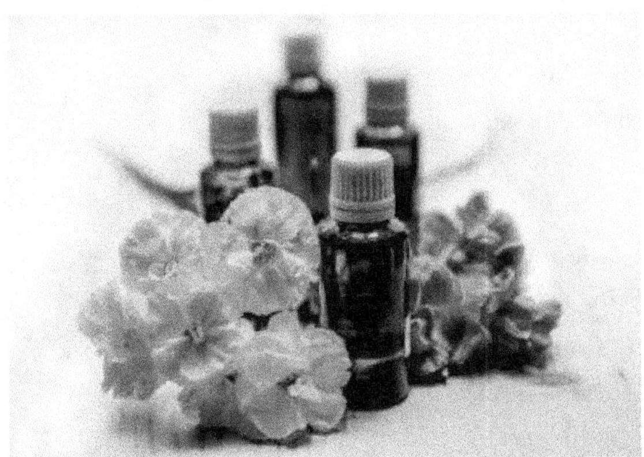

Carrot Seed (Daucus carota)

This is also known as wild carrot. It helps to revitalize the scalp.

Cedarwood (Cedrus atlantica)

This is an essential oil that can help treat dandruff and also promote hair growth. Do not use this oil if pregnant.

Chamomile, Roman (Chamaemelum nobile)

This is a great essential oil for all skin conditions form head to toe. It helps promote healthy hair and scalp.

Clary Sage (Salvia sclarea)

This essential oil is often used to help thinning hair, promote a healthy scalp, fight dandruff, and control oils produced from the sabaceous gland. Do not use if pregnant. It doesn't mix when if you use before you drink alcohol.

Cypress (Cupressus sempervirens)
This oil is used to balance the skin and scalp. It helps to reduce sebum from overactive glands, and regulates the sebum production.

Helichrysum (Helichrysum angustifolium)

This will help with extremely dry scalp.

Lavender (Lavandula angustifolia)

This is an all-purpose essential oil that is good for a skin types. It is often added to shampoos and rinses for dandruff.

Lemon (Citrus limon)

This helps to regulate oily skin and scalp. This can speed a sun burn if used right before going outside.

Patchouli (Pogostemon cablin)

This oil is used often in aromatherapy for hair care, oily hair and skin, and it is also good in treating dandruff.

Rosemary (Rosmarinus officinalis)

This essential oil comes highly recommended for regulating sebum production, stimulating the scalp, helping with thinning hair, ,promoting hair growth, lice, and dandruff. However, it is to be avoided if you are epileptic or suffer from hypertension.

Tea Tree (Melaleuca alternifolia)

This is good for treating dandruff and lice.

Thyme (Thymus vulgaris)

This is another essential oil that can help treat lice. It is also good for regulating oily skin and scalp. This one is however needs to be avoided in cases of hypertension, and pregnancy.

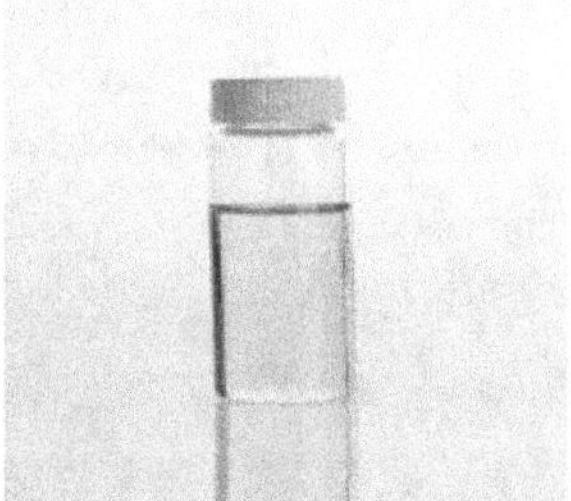

Ylang Ylang (Cananga odorata)

It helps to stimulate hair growth and makes a good ingredient for hair rinses.
As you can see, there are a lot of essential oils you can tailor to your specific needs in terms of hair care. All of the hair care products you tend to buy in the store cannot do that. They are made for a general hair problem and not an individual.

Chapter 2 - Shampoos

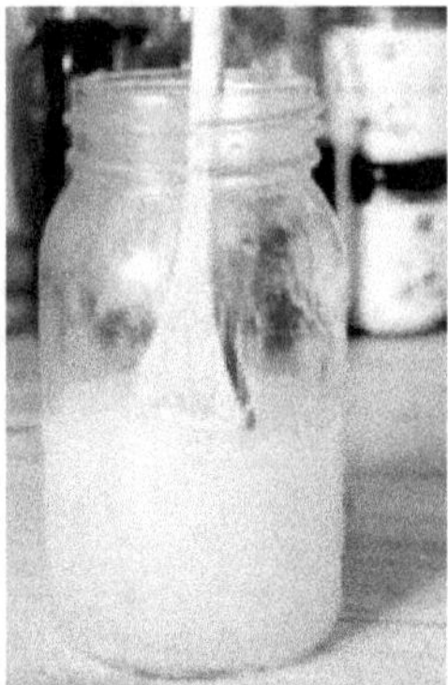

From the most expensive to the ones that only cost a few dollars, all shampoos have chemicals in them that your hair does not need. I will list over a few of these here:

Parabens

These can mimic estrogen, which leads to an imbalance of this hormone in the system and increase the risk of breast cancer. Other names for Parabens are methylparaben, propylparaben, isoparaben, and butylparaben.

Pthalates

This is an ingredient found in items with fragrances that can trigger respiratory problems such as asthma and bronchitis.

1,4-diaxane

This is classified as an animal carcinogen. The FDA, however, allows this compound in shampoos, facial cleansers, and toothpaste. It can also be found in organic products. There are more than 56 ingredients that are related to this compound some of these include:

-sodium laureth sulfate
-sodium myreth sulfate
-polyethylene glycol
-ingredients ending in xynol, ceteareth, and oleth.

Diethanolamine (DEA)

This is an ever-present elmulsifier. Emulsifiers keep the other ingredients in a recipe blended. Up to two-thirds of the products with this chemical in it do not rinse cleanly, leaving DEA to linger on the skin and cause irritation. Cancer, more specifically lung and liver, have been reported, but only if it is a high dose. Other names for this chemical are:

-cocamide DEA
-DEA-cetyl phosphate
-olemide DEA

Formaldehyde

Yes, this is the compound used in preserving human remains and biological specimens. It is often used to smooth hair and skin in soaps and shampoos. It may make you nauseous, cough and can also trigger asthma. They are sneaky with this one, often calling it FRP or some of these names:

-quaternium-15
-dimethyl-dumethyl (DMDM) hydantoin
-imidazolidinyl urea
-sodium hydroxymethylglycinate
Making your own hair care products takes all of these chemicals out of the equation.

You will need a few things to get started making your own shampoo. You probably have these in your kitchen already.

Food Scale

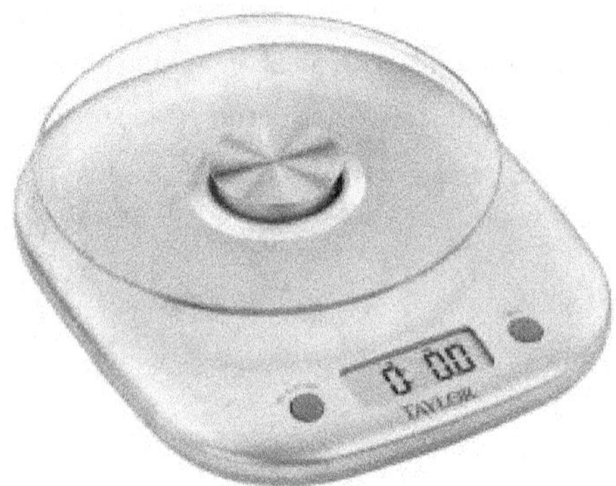

You will be measuring the soap that goes into your shampoo.

Melt and pour soap or Doctor's Bronner's bar soap

You can find melt and pour soap in any craft store, but if you're not comfortable using it, you can purchase Doctor Bronner's Castile Soaps. They do not have the chemicals above.

Empty Shampoo Bottle

You can use any you already have at hand. Just make sure it's rinsed really well.

Blender

This will mix all the ingredients of the shampoo together.

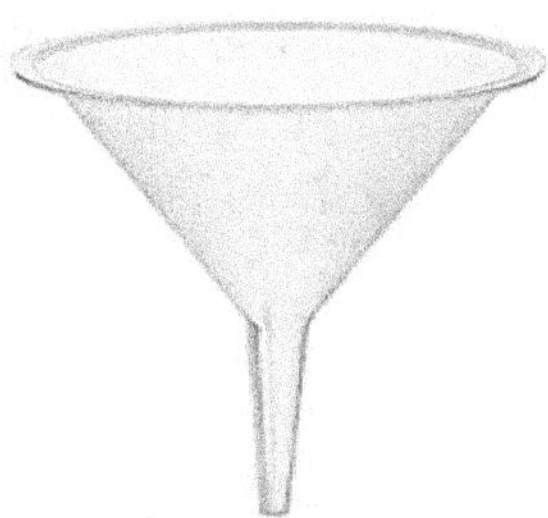

Funnel

This will help you put the shampoo in the bottle of your choice.

Label

This is to label your shampoo and include the ingredients you used to make it.

Oils

Here is a short list of oils commonly used to make homemade shampoo:

Coconut Oil

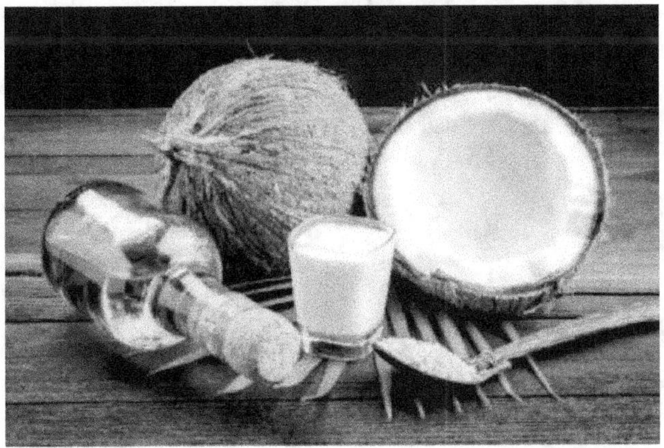

This is rich in minerals and vitamins to nourish your skin. It can also help with frizzing. You will need to get the fractionated version of this oil as the more commonly used version of this oil hardens in temperatures of 76 degrees and below.

Olive oil

This is not the Extra Virgin, but the first press. This oil is darker. Olive oil contains high amounts of vitamin E which is good for the scalp and hair.

Jojoba oil

More a wax than an oil, but it is an oil when in room temperature. This is the closest thing to the sebum your glands produce and can help to bring moisture to hair and a balance to the natural oils in your scalp.

Basic Recipe

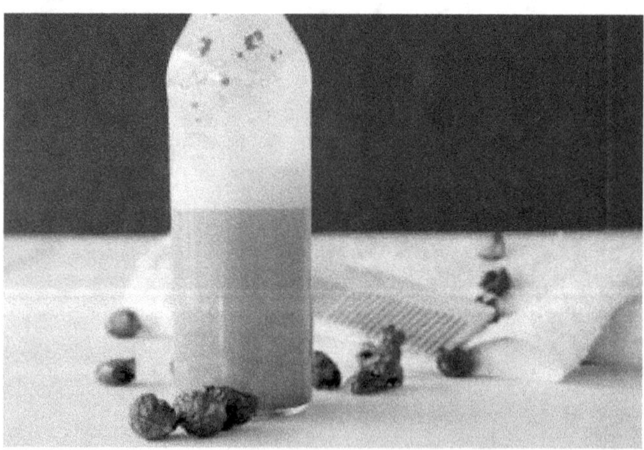

There is a simple recipe for making homemade soap:

4 ounces of Melt and pour or Doctor Bronner's bar soap
1/4 oil

Boiled or filtered water.

50 drops of essential oil

- Grate the soap into a blender.
- Add the oil
- Mix on blend
- Slowly add up to 3/4 cup of water while it is blending.
- Switch to liquify.
- Funnel into the shampoo bottle you are going to use.

If you feel the shampoo is too thick, you can add more water. The shampoo will separate, if you don't use it for a while. This is normal as there are no emulsifiers to keep it from doing so. Because there are no phosphates, it may not lather up as you expect shampoo to do. This is also normal. Your hair is still getting clean, just without extra bubbles.

Dry Scalp I

1/4 Cup Jojoba Oil

10 Drops Carrot Essential Oil

15 Drops Lavender Essential Oil

15 Helichrysum Essential oil

10 Drops Cedarwood Essential Oil

Dry Scalp II

1/4 Cup Coconut Oil

10 Drops Rosemary Essential Oil

15 Drops Cypress Essential Oil

15 Drops Chamomile, Roman Essential Oil

10 Drops Clary sage Essential oil

Dandruff Shampoo

1/4 Cup Olive oil

10 Drops Cedarwood Essential Oil

10 Drops Patchouli Essential Oil

15 Drops Cypress Essential Oil

15 Drops Lavender Essential Oil

Moisturizing Scalp Treatment

2 Eggs (Yes eggs)

10 Drops of Lavender Essential Oil

15 Drops Carrot Essential Oil

15 Drops Helichrysum Essential Oil

- Mix the essential oils, set aside
- Whisk the eggs
- Whisk the essential oils into the eggs.

How to use:

1. Working into damp hair and cover with shower cap.
2. Leave in for twenty minutes
3. Shampoo with dandruff shampoo
4. Use following vinegar rinse.

Vinegar Rinse I

2 Tablespoons Apple Cider Vinegar, unfiltered.

2 Cups water

6 Drops Ylang Ylang Essential Oil

6 Drops Cypress Essential Oil

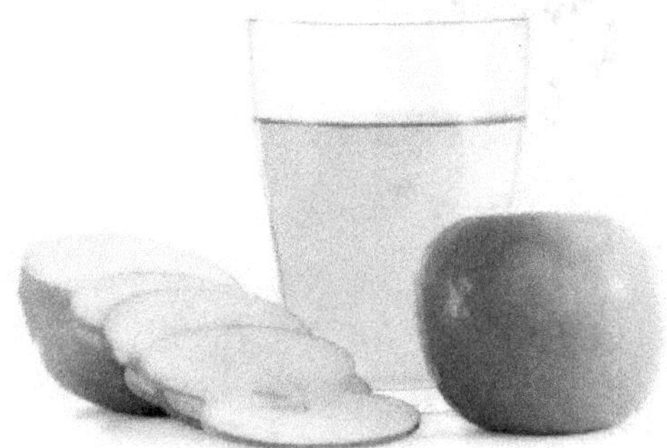

- Mix the essential oils
- Add them to the Apple cider vinegar
- Mix well before adding water. The vinegar not only helps to condition the scalp, but as an emulsifier for the essential oils so they mix better with the water.

How to use:

1. Tilt head backwards in shower or tub.
2. Starting with the front-most hair line, slowly pour the solution so that it soaks into the hair.
3. Use a comb to make sure it evenly distributes on the scalp.
4. Dry and style hair as normal.

Oily Hair

Over washing is one of the many causes of oily scalp and hair. One shouldn't really wash their hair more than three times a week, but most wash daily to get the right style before going to work or out for the evening. Having a naturally oily complexion can normally mean your scalp is oily as well. One has to strike the perfect balance of essential oils in their shampoo and lighter oils in the mix so as not to make it worse.

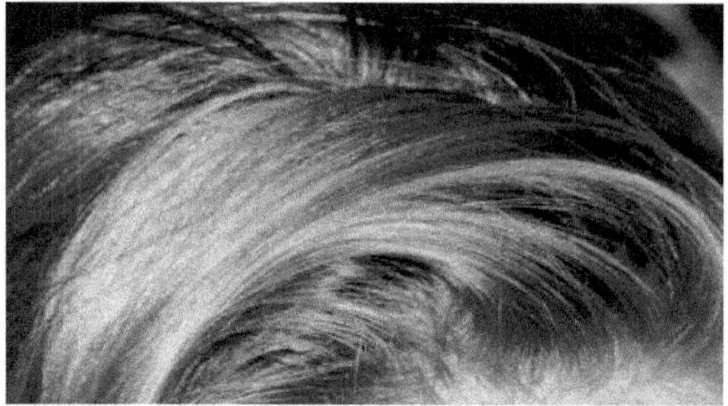

Oils

Sweet Almond Oil

This is a light oil that is packed with the minerals you hair needs without adding to the oily feel of the other oils above.

Apricot Kernel Oil

This has many of the properties of Sweet Almond and thus is a good substitute if you are allergic to tree nuts.

Grapeseed oil

This oil is perhaps the better of the three on this list, but it is a bit more pricey. It provides nutrients to condition the hair and scalp as well as feed it to insure its health.

Essential Oils

There isn't much to add to the list, but there is three more you can add to the mix for helping with excess sebum.

Geranium (Pelargonium graveolens)

This essential oil comes in handy for those with an oily scalp. It helps to curve oils.

Grapefruit (Citrus x paradisi)

This helps to grow the hair. It helps to stem oils created by the skin and scalp.

West Indian Bay (Pimenta racemosa)

This is a scalp stimulant and make a good rinse for dandruff and greasy hair. It also promotes hair growth. Use in small doses and not very often. Since it isn't a more commonly known essential oil, it may be a bit pricey.

Oily Hair I

1/4 Cup Sweet Almond oil
10 Drops Grapefruit Essential Oil
10 Drops Geranium Essential Oil
15 Drops Lavender Essential Oil
15 Drops Cypress Essential Oil

Oily Hair II

1/4 Cup Grapeseed Oil
10 Drops West Indian Bay Essential Oil
10 Drops Thyme Essential Oil
15 Drops Rosemary Essential Oil
15 Drops Carrot Essential Oil

Dry Shampoo

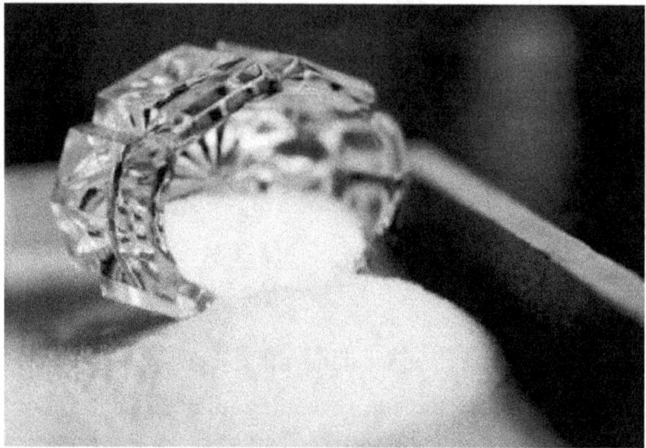

These are "shampoos" that are designed to absorb excess oils in the scalp and used as a stop gap between shampoo sessions:

1. Lightly dab a small amount along part lines.
2. Shake the hair from the root to allow the dry shampoo to fall to the scalp.
3. Take a brush and brush out as much of the hair as possible.

There are one of two things you will need for the dry shampoo:

• Corn starch for light hair
• Cocoa for brown/darker hair.

Dry Shampoo I

1 cup Corn Starch or Cocoa

2 Tablespoons Sweet Almond Oil

6 Drops Lavender Essential Oil

3 Drops Carrot Seed Essential Oil

3 Drops Grapefruit Essential oil

Dry Shampoo II

1 cup Corn Starch or Cocoa

2 Tablespoons of Grapeseed

4 Drops Cedarwood Essential Oil

2 West Indian Bay Essential Oil

4 Drops Cypress Essential Oil

- Mix the oils together
- Mix the dry ingredient into the oils.
- Place the shampoo in a tightly lidded container.

Chapter 3 - Conditioner

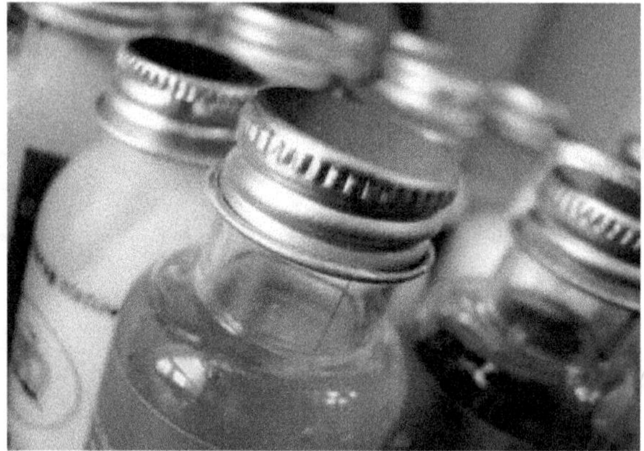

First you shampoo your hair to cleanse it of dirt, sweat, and grit. Then you need to condition it to keep it healthy and strong to prevent breaking. There are typically three types of conditioning:

1. Leave-in
2. Rinse-out
3. Hair mask

The only problem with the second one is that, when you rinse it, you wash most, if not all of it out of your hair, not leaving in enough time to condition the hair or scalp. If it does stay in long enough, it can weigh down the hair.

Leave-in conditioners, sometimes called rinses, are light and designed to stay in the hair, providing extra moisture. This sounds like a good idea, but one good rain and it rinses out, especially if you've done you hair that day.

Hair masks are the type of conditioning masks that stay in for about twenty minutes and then you can wash it out as normal with shampoo.

This are great for infusing your hair with the proteins and minerals you hair needs to get its shine and health back from the abuse everyday styling can do to it. Since these are more intense, by way of conditioning, it isn't recommended you use hair masks no more than once or twice a week, spacing it out by four days.

Moisturizing your hair will help prevent split ends, drying, and breaking. It will also keep your scalp moisturized and healthy, promoting healthy hair as it grows from the shaft. A healthy scalp leads to healthy hair. Here are a few ways you can condition your scalp and hair.

Vinegar Rinse I

2 Cups Water
2 Tablespoons Apple Cider Vinegar unfiltered
6 Drops Ylang Ylang Essential Oil
6 Drops Grapefruit Essential Oil

Vinegar Rinse II

2 Cups Water
2 Tablespoons Apple Cider Vinegar unfiltered
3 Drops Sandalwood Essential Oil
5 Drops Lavender Essential Oil
4 Drops Cypress Essential Oil

Hair Masks

This may sound a bit weird, but hair masks work like facials for your hair and scalp. They nourish your hair, can repair the damage done through styling, and even promote hair growth if your hair is thinning. Hair masks can also provide much needed moisture to your scalp and hair, making it less frizzy and more manageable.

Avocado and Egg Mask (dry scalp)

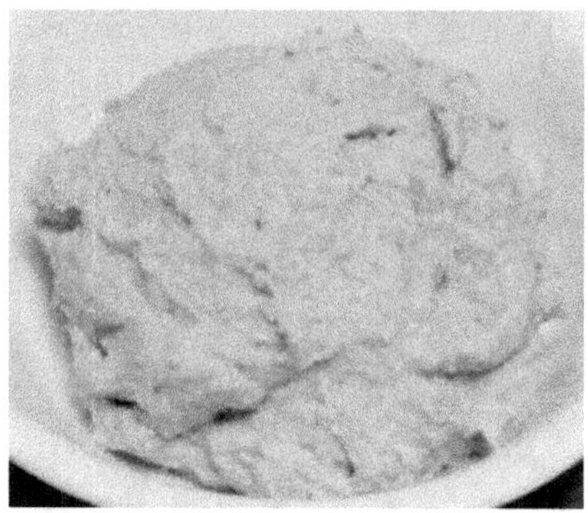

Eggs are an excellent source of protein and avocados provide your hair with oils that can help condition it.

1/2 and Avocado
2 Egg yolks
10 Drops Carrot Essential oil
10 Drops Rosemary Essential oil
20 Drops Lavender Essential oil
10 Drops Sandalwood Essential oil

- Mix the essential oils separately
- Mash the avocado
- Mix the egg yolks into the avocado well
- Mix in the essential oils

How to use:

1. Work into damp hair.
2. Leave in for 15-20 minutes
3. Rinse out in the shower
4. Apply one of the vinegar rinses

Honey and Yogurt Mask (dry scalp)

Honey is sticky and can be a pain to get out of anything once it's been applied, but when you mix with other ingredients, it becomes easy to rinse out.

1 tsp olive oil
1 tsp honey, preferably raw and unfiltered
1/4 Cup yogurt
10 Drops Patchouli Essential oil
10 Drops of Cypress Essential oil
5 Drops of Clary Sage Essential oil

- Mix the essential oil separately from the other ingredients
- Mix the honey and olive oil
- Add the essential oils to the honey and olive oil
- Whisk them into the yogurt

Use as directed for the egg and avocado recipe.

Avocado and Egg (Oily Scalp) I

1/2 and Avocado
2 Egg yolks
10 Drops Lemon Essential oil
10 Drops Cypress Essential oil
15 Drops Ylang Ylang Essential Oil
Directions as above.

Honey Yogurt Mask (Oily Scalp) II

1 tsp olive oil

1 tsp honey, preferably raw and unfiltered

1/4 Cup yogurt

15 Drops Grapefruit Essential oil

5 Drops Rosemary Essential oil

10 Drops Sandalwood Essential oil

5 Drops Carrot Seed Essential oil

Follow Direction as above

Maintenance Mask

This is a simple mask to keep your hair shiny and healthy.

1 tsp olive oil

1 tsp honey, preferably raw and unfiltered

1/4 Cup yogurt

10 Drops Ylang Ylang Essential oil

10 Drops Carrot Seed Essential oil

10 Drops Cypress Essential oil

Follow directions as above.

Chapter 4 - Hair styling products

Now, we're getting to the crux of the matter. It's one thing to make natural products for your hair to condition and clean it, but it is exponentially harder to find all natural products to style and treat your hair. Don't worry. Here are some recipes to get you started.

Mousses and Gels

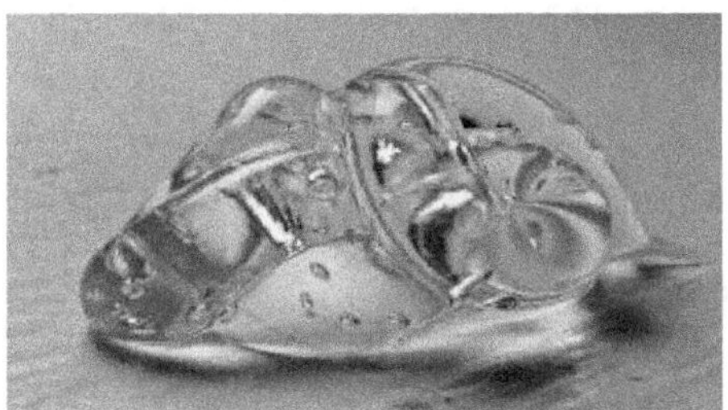

These are the two most popular methods of styling hair. They both help to retain you style, but their difference in consistency means you can't use them for all types of hair.

Mousse

This is typically used for people with naturally curly hair to keep the curls and manage the frizz without compromising the natural bounce of the curls. This also works well for permed curls.

Gels

This product is mostly used for straight hair when trying to maintain a curly style or to keep up a certain look. People with curly hair use it to crunch their curls to make them tight.

Hair Pomade/Balm

This product looks like a cream and is usually sold in either tubes or a container resembling facial cream. It is used to smooth out frizz and make the hair a little more manageable. It doesn't take much to get the results you need. A small pea-sized amount will do the trick. Rub it in your hands and then work it into your hair.

Hair Mousse Basic Recipe

No matter the essential oils you add to your homemade mousse, the basic recipe is the same.

1/2 Cup Shea Butter (moisturizing for the hair)
1/4 Cup Coconut oil (Nutrients for the hair)
1/4 cup Olive oil

• Melt the Shea Butter with the Coconut oil and whip it with a hand mixer for ten minutes
• Add the essential oils while mixing
• Drizzle in the olive oil while mixing
• Add the finished product in a tightly lidded container.

Dry Hair Mousse

10 Drops Carrot Seed Essential oil
20 Drops Lavender Essential oil
20 Drops Cypress Essential oil
20 Drops Roman Chamomile Essential oil
10 Drops Tea Tree Essential oil

Oily Hair Mousse

20 Drops Grapefruit essential oil
10 Drops of Rosemary Essential oil
10 Drops of Ylang Ylang Essential oil
20 Drops of Geranium Essential oil
10 Drops of Sandalwood Essential oil
10 Drops of Lavender Essential oil

Basic Gel Recipe

1/4 tsp pure, unflavored gelatin
1/2 Cup Hot water

- Bring the water to boiling
- Stir in the gelatin.
- When it cools to warm, add your essential oils.

For Dry Hair

10 Drops Cypress Essential oil
10 Drops Lavender Essential oil
5 Drops Helichrysum Essential oil
5 Drops Clary Sage Essential oil

For Oily Hair

10 Drops Grapefruit Essential oil
10 Drops Carrot Seed Essential oil
10 Drops Geranium Essential oil

Hair Pomade/Balm Basic Recipe

1 Ounce Organic Beeswax

1.5 Ounces of Shea Butter

2 Ounces Jojoba Oil

- Melt the beeswax in a double boiler
- Melt in the Shea Butter
- Stir in the Jojoba oil
- As it is cooling, add the essential oils

Dry Hair

10 Drops Patchouli Essential oil

10 Drops Ylang Ylang Essential oil

10 Drops of Roman Chamomile Essential oil

Oily Hair

10 Drops Grapefruit Essential oil

10 Drops Cypress Essential oil

10 Drops Carrot Seed Essential oil

Hair Spray

You've got the mousse, the gel, and the pomade. All you need is the hairspray to keep it all in place. There are two basic recipes you can use, one with sugar and one without.

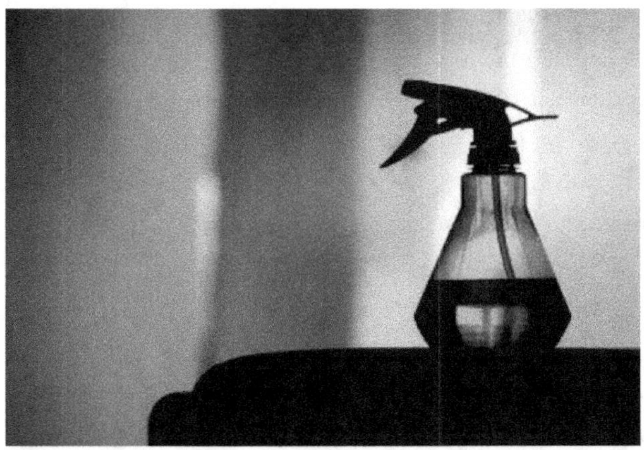

1 Whole Organic Orange (for dark hair) or Organic Lemon (for light hair)

2 Cups distilled or filtered water

2-3 Tbsp High Proof Vodka (or other clear alcohol)

- Wedge the fruit and place it in a pot.
- Add the water and bring to a boil
- Reduce the liquid to half by boiling it down.
- Strain through a cheesecloth to get all of the juice out of the fruit.
- You should have one cup by this time.
- Funnel into a spray bottle after it has cooled.
- Add your essential oils until they are mixed in well.

Sugar Hairspray

1.5 Cups filtered water

2 tablespoons white sugar

1 tablespoon high proof clear alcohol, like vodka

10-15 Drops of essential oils

- Boil water to dissolve the sugar
- Add essential oils to the alcohol
- Add the alcohol solution to the sugar water
- Shake well.
- Adjust the sugar level to increase or decrease the hold of the hairspray.

You can add the following essential oils to the hairspray. The only trick is to wait until the solutions have cooled and shake well.

Luster

20 Drops Ylang Ylang
10 Drops Carrot Seed Essential oil

Moisture

20 Drops Lavender Essential oil
10 Roman Chamomile Essential oil
You can mix and match essential oils to have different aromas for your hairspray.

Chapter 5 - Thinning Hair

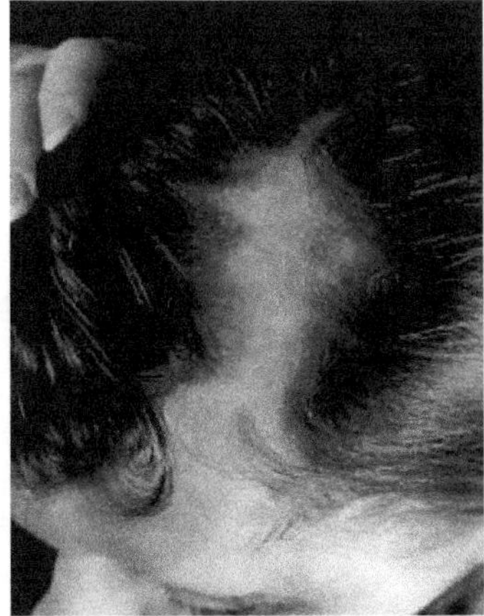

There are several reasons for thinning hair and hair loss. Heredity, stress, and malnutrition are three known causes, but there are some recipes you can make to help keep from losing more, and in some cases, grow some of it back.

The following recipes should be used three times a week.

There really aren't essential oils to add to this list. So I will list the ones from the previous chapter:

Carrot Seed
Cedarwood
Chamomile, Roman
Clary Sage
Lavender
Rosemary
West Indian Bay

This is a basic base to use for the essential oils.

- 4 tsp Jojoba Oil
- 4 tsp Coconut Oil

To Use:

If you are bald:

1. Massage into scalp and let it settle into the scalp
2. Wash with one of the shampoos a previous chapter.
3. Follow up with a vinegar rinse and work it into the scalp.

If you have a thinning spot:

1. Part the hair
2. With your finger tips, work the recipe into the part.
3. Repeat until the thinning spot is worked with the recipe.
4. Place shower cap on your head.
5. Leave in for 15 minutes
6. Wash hair with one of the shampoos in a previous chapter.
7. Use a vinegar rinse.

Recipe I

3 Drops Lavender Essential oil

2 Drops Rosemary Essential oil

2 Drops West Indian Bay Essential oil

Recipe II

3 Drops Roman Chamomile Essential oil
2 Drops Thyme Essential oil
2 Drops Carrot Seed Essential oil

Recipe III

2 Drops Clary Sage Essential oil
2 Drops Cedarwood Essential oil
2 Drops Lavender Essential oil

Chapter 6 - Healthy Hair From the Inside

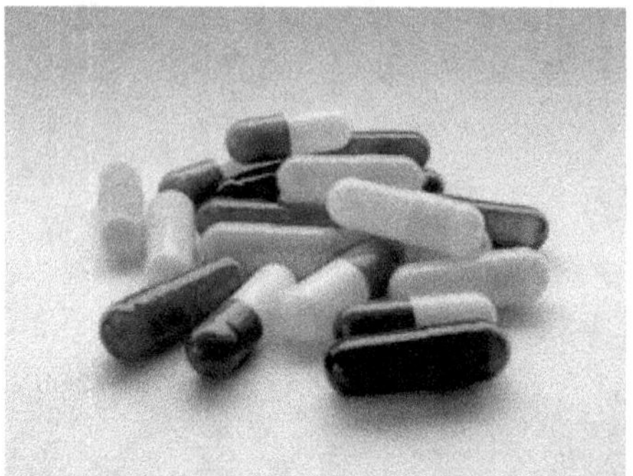

We've discussed how to tackle making your hair and scalp on the surface. In this chapter, I will go over some vitamins, minerals, and herbal supplements to help you get stronger and healthier hair from the inside.

Vitamins and minerals

Fish oils

This is high in Omega-3 fatty acids. It helps thicken the hair, and promote a healthy scalp.

Zinc

Zinc is instrumental to helping prevent the regression of hair follicles. It also helps to heal damaged and irritated follicles. Fun fact: Some people who suffer from alopecia have a zinc deficiency.

B-Complex, Biotin and B5

B-complex, in general, promotes healthy hair, but biotin and panatothenic acid (b5) help to speed healing of damaged hair from over styling.

Vitamin C

This helps slow the aging of the hair, preventing the hair from turning gray.

Iron

Adding iron-rich foods like Swiss chard, collard greens, egg yolks, beef, spinach, and beans, preferably navy and black beans.

Vitamin D

A deficiency of this vitamin can actually speed hair loss. On warm days, you can sit outside in the sun for about 15 minutes to absorb your daily dose. During the winter months, an herbal based Vitamin D is recommended with an intake of 10,000 units daily.

Herbals

Aloe Vera

This juice is packed with the vitamins and minerals to help promote healthy hair and hair growth.

Horsetail

This is a highly recommended herb for strengthening the hair and promoting hair growth. It's also good for strong nails, too.

Kelp

This herb has natural minerals that can help thicken and strengthen the hair. Combined with horsetail, it's a potent one-two punch for hair health and growth.

Conclusion

This is just to get you started. There are many more recipes to experiment with and try. There are online forums you can join which can help you make you own combinations and further tailor your hair health to your personal body's metabolism. I hope this book has helped answer many of your questions. Until next time...

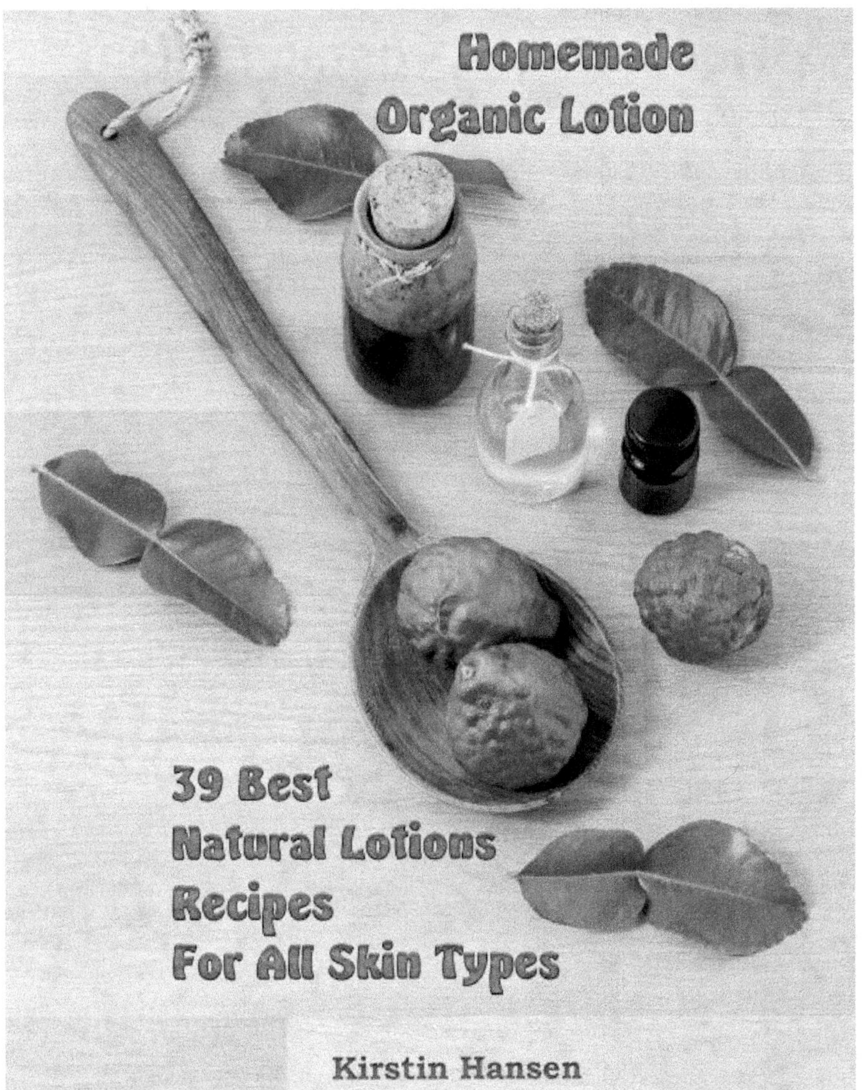

Homemade
Organic Lotion

39 Best
Natural Lotions
Recipes
For All Skin Types

Kirstin Hansen

Homemade Organic Lotion:

39 Best Natural Lotions Recipes for All Skin Types

Introduction

How much sense does it make to water a plastic tree? In my mind, not much. Most of what I've come across in the world of body lotions have been synthetic scientifically engineered chemicals.

Some people find such things to be fantastically useful advances in science. While I feel respect for what people today are able to do and create I remain in favor of a more natural approach to life.

It is a difficult market for those who share my sense of connection to an innate naturalistic method of living. Much of what is sold to us is composed of again, synthetic, man-engineered items. This is significant in the sense that often times such things are composed of individually toxic parts, yet as a whole avoid a dangerous level of toxicity.

The same can be said of products in the cosmetic industry. Frequently products contain elements which are not only insufficient at solving the problem they claim to, but are dangerous and harmful to the skin. Most of the time there are only trace amounts of these hazardous chemical compounds so the damage frequently occurs in the long run following extended use.

For the aforementioned reasons I strictly prefer natural lotions as they are composed of nonhazardous, naturally occurring substances. That is not to say that there are not harmful or poisonous substances that occur naturally in our environment. Yet when it comes to taking care of our skin it seems sensible to me to take advantage of the gentle solutions offered by the earth.

Natural body lotions have a greater success rate when it comes to fulfilling their promise. In most cases the particular skin type is not important as all skin benefits from some key vitamins and topical mixtures.

There are also less cases of people having adverse reactions to natural body lotions. They do not contain alcohol, which severely dries the skin, and they maintain a soothing moisturizing factor that nourishes the skin.

Everyone is entitled to their own opinion but for those who are looking to take the best care of themselves they can, I say do it the natural way.

Chapter 1 – Before You Begin

Understanding Skin Types

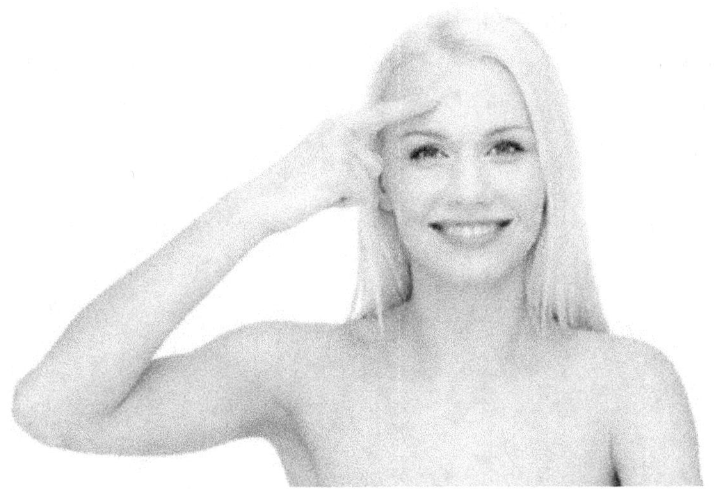

Everybody is physically unique. In your shape, size, and composition. Everything about you is unique exactly to you—including your skin. One thing about buying lotions at the store that can be difficult is trying to find one bottle of lotion that is made for your exact skin type and meets all of your skin care needs.

Not all lotions are created equally, and with the mass marketing of brands, many skin types can get over-looked. Or, if you don't have normal skin, you may end up paying an arm and a leg for specialty lotions designed for oily or dry skin and price marked way more than they are worth.

Some lotions or creams can run upward of forty dollars. What are you paying for? More often than not, you're paying for the brand name or some expensive lab-created ingredient that does exactly the same thing as its organic counterparts.

By making your own lotion at home, you can guarantee that you create a product for the skin you have, and the skin you want. This will allow you to reap the benefits of having healthy, moisturized, hydrated skin and give you the opportunity to add some protective ingredients to prevent against environmental irritation.

While every person is unique, there are several basic categories of skin types that people fall into. Typically, after puberty you should have a pretty good idea of where you fall on the scale. If you aren't sure or if you just want to double check, read through the descriptions below and find the one that fits best with how you would describe your skin.

There are four major types of skin:

- Dry
- Normal
- Combination
- Oily

Each skin type has their own traits and attributes that can help you identify which type you have. You may not have all the traits of a certain skin type, or you may find that you have some from multiple skin type descriptions. Some skin can fall into more than one type.

Read through the descriptions and if you match more than one skin type, rank them based on how many traits you have in each category. Chances are if you only have one or two traits from a single category, then it is not enough to classify you as that primary skin type.

When making your lotion, go off your primary skin type for the area of your body that you want to use the lotion on. If your face identifies as one skin type but your body is another, then you may need to make two lotions: one for your face and one for your body. That way your skin gets the best treatment based on the primary type it aligns with.

Dry skin if you suffer from dry skin you can identify this condition by the following traits:

- Small pores which are almost unnoticeable
- Red, patchy skin
- Itchy skin
- Cracked skin
- Peeling skin

Dry skin can be a result of genetics, medication, or a medical condition. Treating dry skin is important to maintain skin elasticity, comfort, and prevent other possible heath conditions.

Normal Skin Normal skin can be identified by the following traits:

- Few imperfections or blemishes
- Small pores which are barely visible
- Minimal sensitivity or no severe sensitivity

Most people will have normal skin after puberty. This has a light, healthy layer of oils that keep the skin lightly moisturized and gives a "radiant" appearance.

Combination Skin Combination skin affects the highest percentage of individuals. Combination skin means having more than one skin type.

Typically, this can be identified if you have patches of dry or oily skin and patches of normal skin. This can look like normal skin with an oily T-zone on your face, or normal skin all over with patches of dry skin on your arms, *etc.*

Traits of Combination Skin are:

- Noticeable or dilated pores

- Blackheads
- "Shiny" or an oily sheen on the skin
- Spots of red, patchy skin

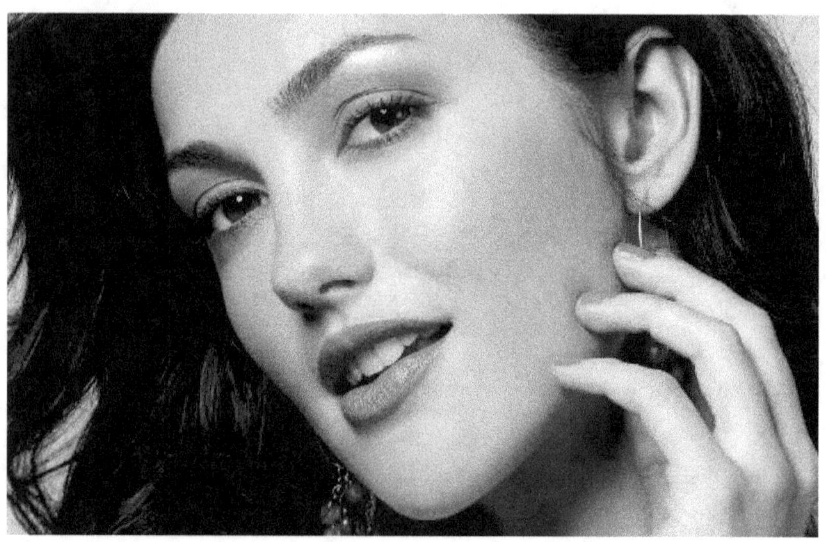

Combination skin can be treated by making two different types of lotion, or by focusing on whichever skin type is more dominant. If your skin is oilier than it is normal or dry, then focus on that skin type.

Oily Skin Oily skin is very common for individuals going through puberty and some adults. This is because the change in hormones can result in the body producing more oil for the skin.

Traits of oily skin are:

- Oversized or enlarged pores
- A thick oily sheen or "shine" to the skin
- Acne, blackheads, and clogged pores
- A feeling of "heaviness" to the skin due to the exaggerated oil production.

If you have oily skin it is important to clean your skin regularly to prevent dirt and grime from getting trapped in the pores. Hydrating the skin can help keep it healthy. Avoid drying out the skin unless you are treating on-the-spot acne. Drying out oily skin too much can result in other skin conditions.

Once you have identified the type of skin you have, it will make the process of selecting what type of lotion to make that much easier. You may find that it is best for you to make multiple lotion types for different areas of the skin.

Base Ingredients of the Lotion.

Lightweight lotion oils: This is best if you are making a lotion for any skin type.

- Olive Oil

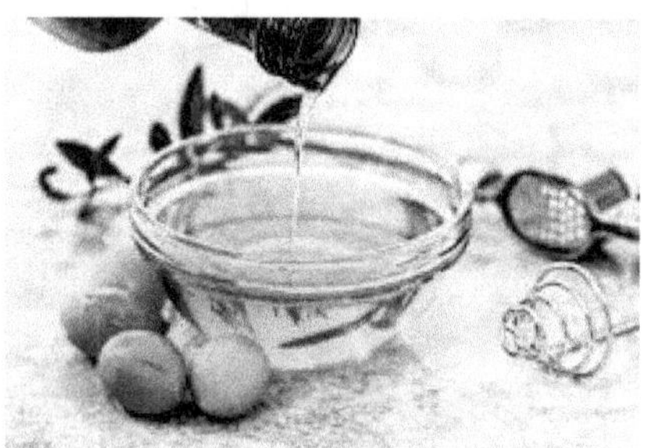

Olive oil has antioxidants and Vitamin E in it to protect your skin from premature aging, ultraviolet rays, and skin damage. It also doesn't clog pores and it enhances exfoliation to clear away dead skin cells. This is great for all skin types.

- Almond Oil

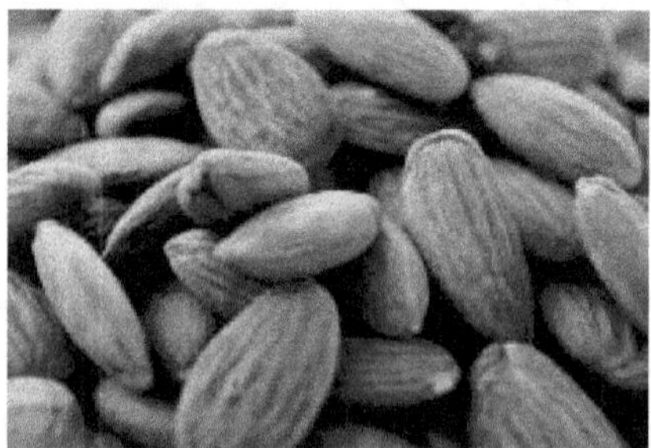

Almond oil is hypoallergenic (provided you do not have a nut allergy ;) it has Vitamin A to help clean the pores, remove dirt, and reduce acne; it can relieve irritation to the skin due to sun exposure; and it can help treat eczema. This is great for normal to dry skin.

- Coconut Oil

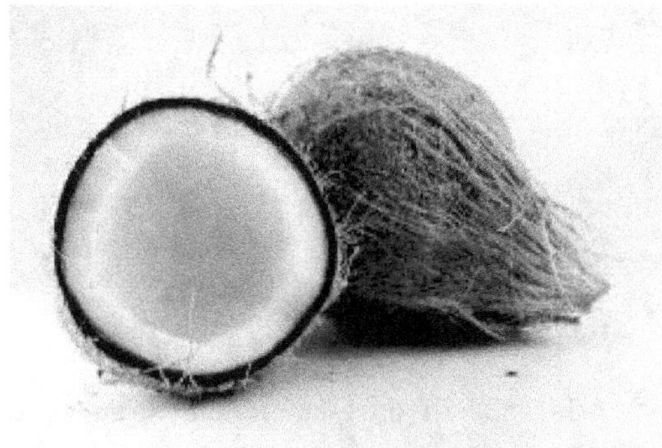

Coconut oil has saturated fats which help retain moisture in the skin. It also has Vitamin E which protects the skin from ultraviolet rays, premature aging, and skin damage. This is great for all skin types.

- Avocado Oil

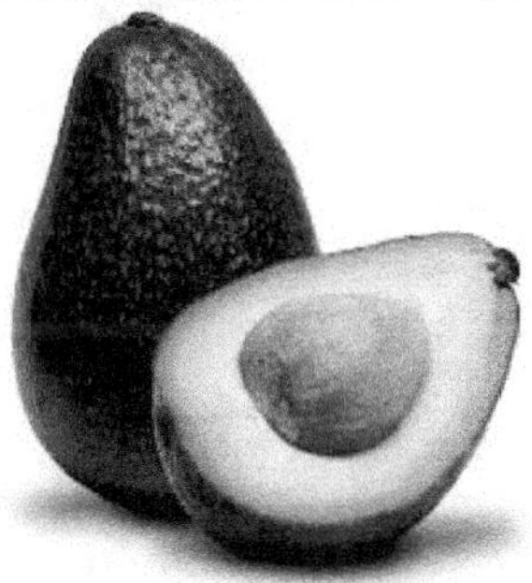

Avocado oil is high in nutrients and vitamin which are valuable to the skin. It enhances the natural ability for the skin to create collagen, which is what retains the skin's elasticity and firmness. The proteins and fats in the oil help keep the skin moisturized which can help treat eczema and other dry skin issues. This is great for normal to dry skin.

- Apricot Oil

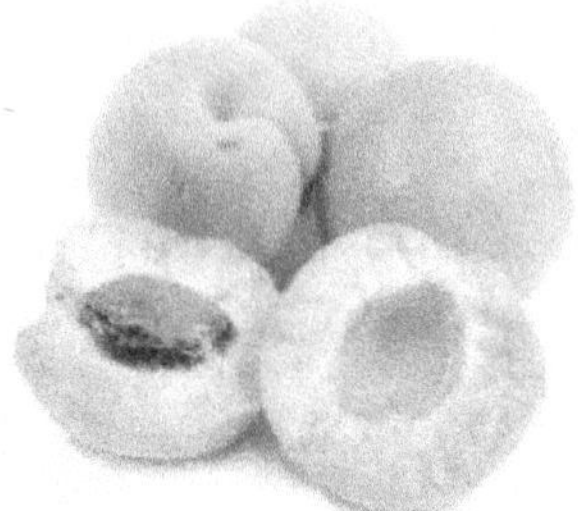

Apricot oil is great for normal skin, oily skin, and hormonal skin. It is gentle and does not leave an oily residue or coat on the skin. Because of this, it is great for the face or oily skin due to its lightness.

Heavy weight butters these are best for body butters or creams for normal to dry skin, or if you want long lasting moisture without needing to reapply.

- Cocoa Butter

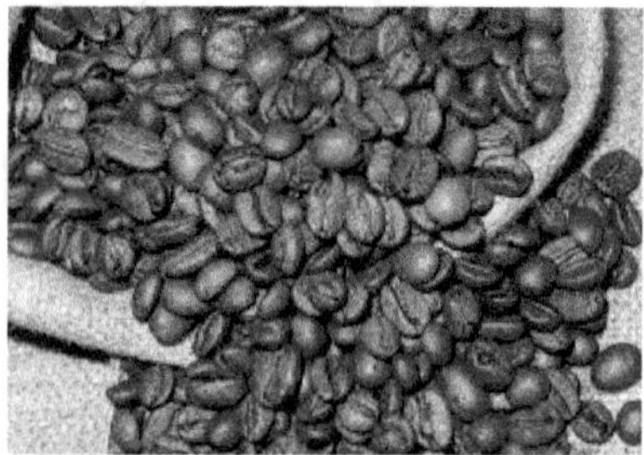

Cocoa butter is a good replacement to use if you have any nut allergies. Cocoa butter is thick, and gentle on the skin. It is pure vegetable fat harvested from the cocoa bean. The fat in cocoa butter helps the skin retain moisture and it works to smooth the skin and has anti-aging properties, as well. It is also rich in antioxidants which protect the skin from damage caused by ultraviolet rays and other external factors that can cause skin irritation or harm.

- Shea Butter

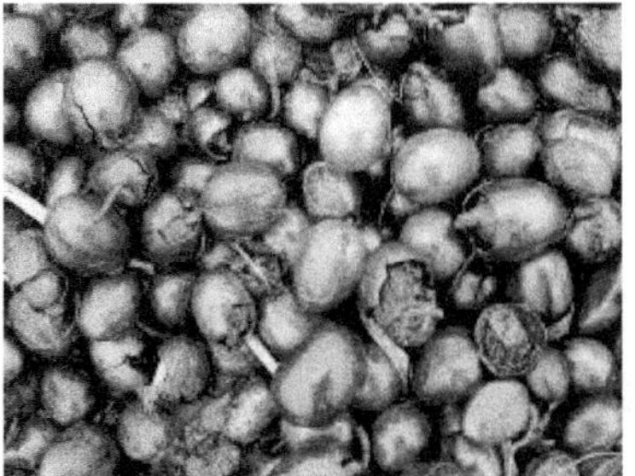

Shea butter is the most common ingredient in heavy weight body butters. Shea butter not only moisturizes skin, but the nutrients and vitamins in it help to restore collagen for skin elasticity. Shea butter also works as an anti-inflammatory for irritated skin, it reduces stretch marks, protects skin from ultraviolet rays, and is gentle enough on the skin that it can be used on babies. If you have nut allergies, don't use Shea butter, but opt for cocoa butter instead.

If you want to make a mid-weight cream, combine one of the lightweight oils with a small amount of one of the butters. This will thicken the lotion just enough to make it a cream, without adding all the weight of a body butter.

Types of Lotion

There are several different types of lotion and each one has its own function and purpose. Based on your skin type, and the needs of your skin that you're hoping your homemade organic lotion will help with, you may need to make a certain kind of lotion or several to meet a variety of needs.

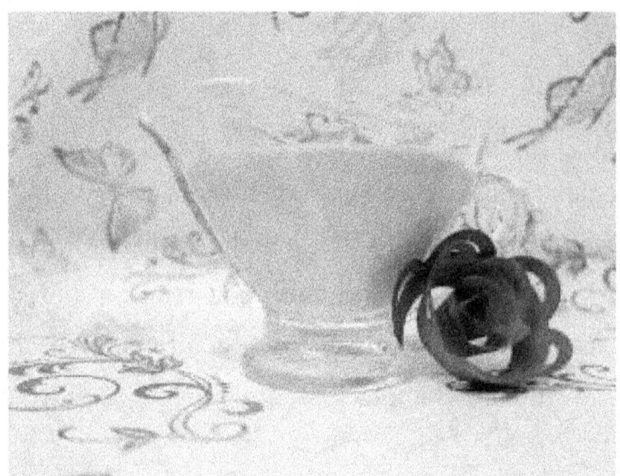

There are two main types of lotion that you can easily make at home:

- Generic lotion
- Body butter

Each type of lotion has a different function and a different base to give it a specific weight. When discussing "weight" as it pertains to a lotion, the weight corresponds with how thick the lotion is. The lighter it is, the faster it absorbs and the more likely you are going to need to reapply it. The thicker it is, the longer it will sit on the skin to moisturize it.

There are pros and cons to each weight, and those will depend on your skin type and your everyday needs.

Lightweight A lightweight lotion is going to have a light oil base and will blend easily into the skin. It will typically absorb right away, or within a few minutes. This can be nice if you can't afford oily or greasy hands or appendages, but it also means you will need to reapply more frequently.

A lightweight lotion is great for people with oily skin who do not need a lot of extra moisturizer, but still want to give their skin the extra nutrients and benefits that come with moisturizing.

Lightweight lotions are also great for hands. Lightweight lotion is good to use for your hands because if you use your hands a lot at work, and depending on what you do, you might not be able to afford oily or greasy hands which can happen if you use a lotion that is too heavy.

Lightweight lotions are also perfect to use on your face because you don't want anything too heavy that could clog your pores and lead to acne. A nice, lightweight lotion will moisturize your skin and help with the appearance of wrinkles as well as preventing breakouts. Although it is a common misconception that oil=acne, moisturized and hydrated skin can actually prevent breakouts. This is because well-moisturized skin has a healthy layer of oil which protects against dryness and dirt which can lead to clogged pores and result in acne. Too much oil can also trap dirt, which is why cleaning and washing your face regularly is important.

Mid-weight A mid-weight lotion is good for normal or combination skin. Combination skin is where you have both oily and normal or dry skin. This can result in specific spots where your skin is oilier—like an oily T-zone.

Mid-weight lotions will absorb into the skin a little more slowly than a lightweight lotion, but won't stay on the skin as long as a heavier butter. This is why having a mid-weight lotion or cream is great for the hands or body.

Heavy weight A heavy weight lotion is also known as a butter or cream. This might be more recognizable as a body butter. Heavy lotions or butter stay on the skin for long periods of time. While this can be troublesome if you have it on your hands because it will leave an oily or greasy residue for a while until it is absorbed completely into the skin, it also works the best because it lasts the longest and provides your skin with long-lasting moisture and hydration.

Body butters or heavy lotions are great for using on the body and extremities such as the arms or legs. It will go on thick and slowly absorb into the skin throughout the day or night (depending on when you put it on.) Heavy lotions or body butters are great for people with dry skin or chronic dry skin because it will provide a layer of moisture on top of the skin while it soaks in. It is also good to use for people with normal or combination skin.

Heavy lotions or butters can be too much for people with oily skin. Adding this additional moisture to already oily skin can result in a greasy feeling, a heaviness to the skin, and clogged pore which can lead to acne.

If you're not sure what skin type you have, you can test each lotion weight on a patch of skin to find out. It is recommended to test on a patch of skin on your arm where it can be easily washed if you do not like the result of the product.

The great thing about making your own lotion is that you can make it to fit your exact skin type.

More details will be provided in Chapters 3 and 4, but it is best to start with the lightweight lotion and then add more ingredients as needed to make it mid-weight (cream) or heavy weight (butter).

Chapter 2 – Lotions for Dry Skin

Pumpkin Spice Lotion

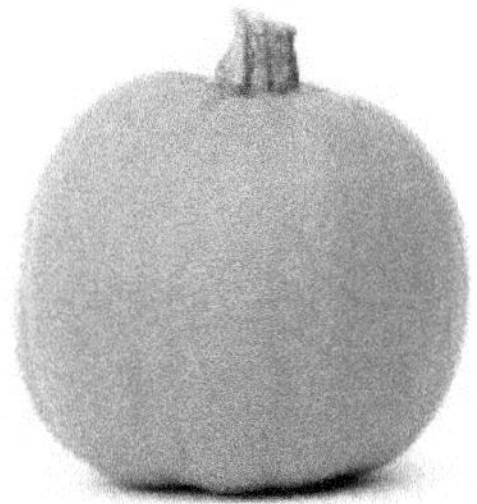

Ingredients:

- 8 ounces of shea butter
- 2 cups of coconut oil
- 20 drops of pumpkin spice essential oil

Directions:

1. Melt the coconut oil with shea butter in a double boiler then remove it from the heat while some soft chunks of butter are still visible.

2. Blend the mix with a stand mixer until it becomes smooth and creamy then add in the essential oil and blend it again.

3. Transfer the lotion into mason jars and secure their lids then allow it to cool down completely.

4. Apply this lotion to your body whenever you desire.

5. This lotion smells heavenly and softens your skin at the same time.

Creamy Coconut Aloe Vera Lotion

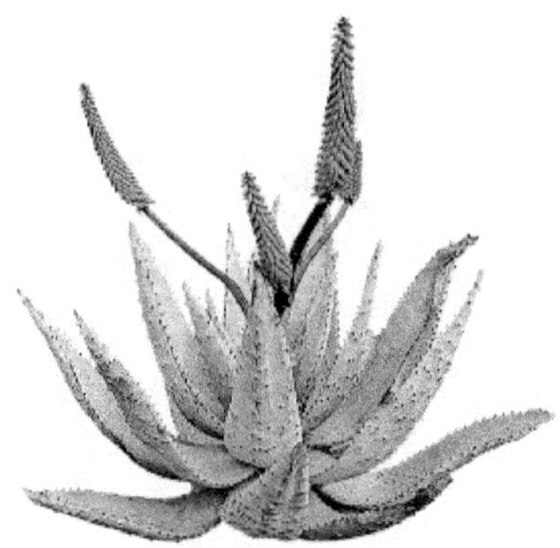

Ingredients:

- ¼ cup of solid coconut oil
- 1 teaspoon of aloe vera gel
- 3 drops of rose essential oil
- 2 drops of lavender essential oil

Directions:

1.	Beat the coconut oil using a hand mixer until it becomes creamy then stir into it the essential oil and aloe vera gel.

2.	Transfer the lotion to a mason jar and seal the lid then use it right away or refrigerate it.

3.	After an eventful day, this lotion will help you relax your sore muscles.

Creamy Jojoba Lotion

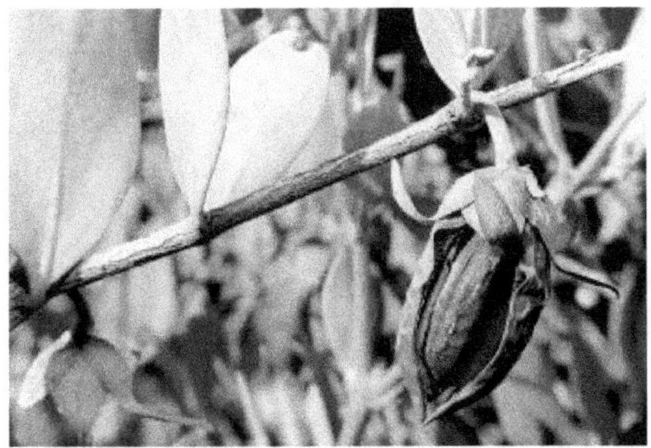

Ingredients:

- 1 cup of cold pressed coconut oil
- 1 cup of pure shea butter
- 2 tablespoons of vegetable glycerin
- 1 tablespoon of jojoba oil

Directions:

1. Combine all the ingredients in a food processor and blend them smooth then transfer the mix to a bowl and refrigerate it until it solidifies.

2. Once the time is up, whip the lotion with a hand mixer until it becomes creamy.

3. Apply this lotion to your body whenever you desire.

4. This lotion is nourishing; it will smoothen and soften your skin.

Grapefruit Body Lotion

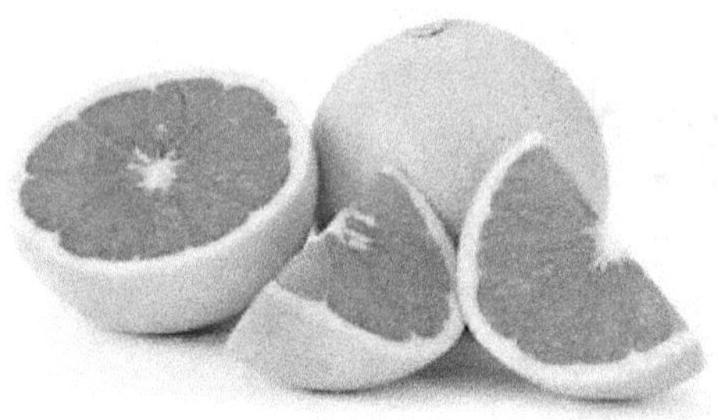

Ingredients:

- ½ cup of coconut oil
- The zest of 1 red grapefruit
- 2 tablespoons of raw shea butter
- 2 teaspoons of tapioca starch
- 2 drops of almond essential oil

Directions:

1.   Combine the coconut oil with shea butter and grapefruit zest in a bowl and beat them for 30 sec on medium then turn it on high and whip it for another 4 min.

2.   Once the time is up, add in the rest of the ingredients and whip them for another 30 sec.

3.   Apply this lotion to your body whenever you desire.

4.   This lotion will nourish and moisturize your skin.

Lavender Arrow Lotion

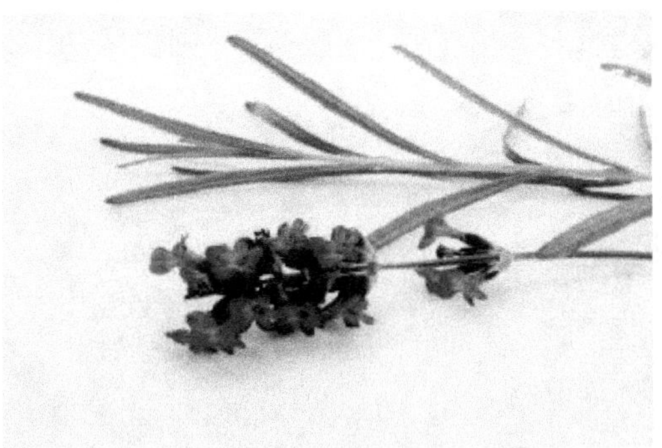

Ingredients:

- 1 cup of coconut oil
- 1 cup of raw shea butter
- 1/3 cup of arrowroot powder
- 100 drops of lavender essential oil

Directions:

1. Combine all the ingredients in a medium bowl and whip them until their soft peaks.

2. Transfer the mix into a mason jar and seal it then use it right away or refrigerate it until ready to use.

3. If you want a creamy lotion that moisturizes your skin without making it greasy, this lotion is perfect for you.

Woodsy Myrrh Lotion

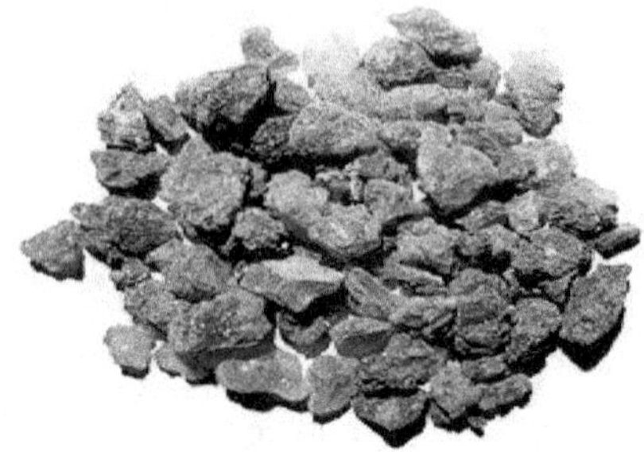

Ingredients:

- ¼ cup of coconut oil
- ¼ cup of raw shea butter
- ¼ cup of olive oil
- ¼ cup of beeswax
- 20 drops of myrrh essential oil
- 20 drops of frankincense essential oil

Directions:

1.   Combine all the ingredients in a double boiler except for the essential oils and stir them until they completely melt.

2.   Remove the mix from the heat and sit in the essential oils then whip them until they become fluffy and creamy.

3.   Transfer the mix into a mason jar and seal it then use it right away or refrigerate it until ready to use.

4.   This lotion with make your skin soft and smooth like a baby's.

Chapter 3 – Lotions for Normal Skin

Minty Aloe Vera Lotion

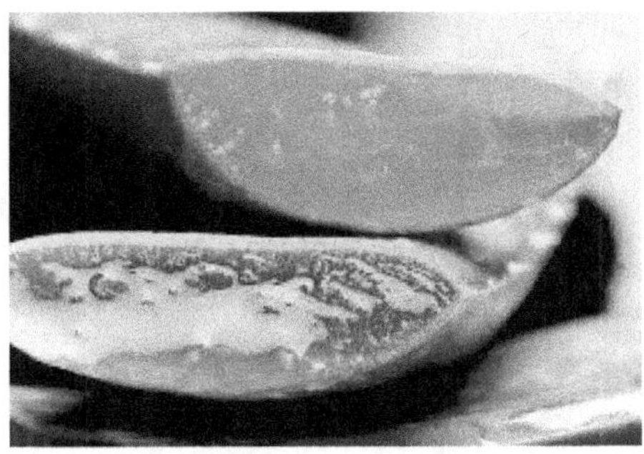

Ingredients:

- ½ cup of aloe vera gel
- ½ cup of coconut oil
- ¼ cup of beeswax, grated
- 1/8 teaspoon of peppermint oil

Directions:

1. Melt the wax with coconut oil in a double boiler then remove it from the heat.

2. Add in the peppermint oil with aloe vera gel and whisk them until they become smooth.

3. Place the lotion in an ice bath and stir it until it becomes creamy and slightly thick then allow it to cool down for 1 h.

4.   Once the time is up, transfer the lotion to a food processor and blend it for 30 sec.

5.   Transfer the mix into a mason jar and seal it then use it right away or refrigerate it until ready to use.

6.   This lotion will be sooth your skin and repairs all the damage that the sun caused to it.

Floral Lotion

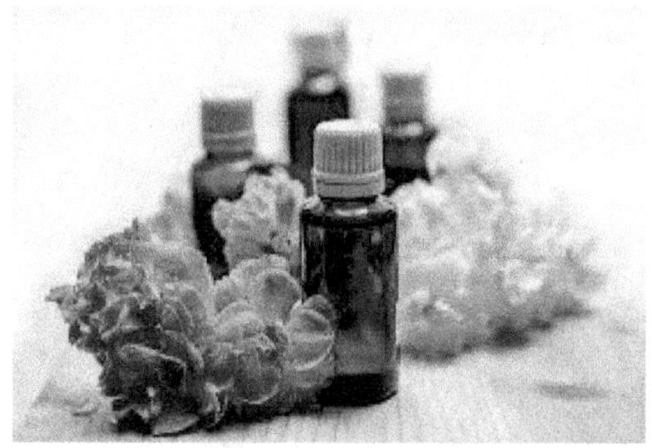

Ingredients:

- ½ cup of orange floral water
- ¾ cup of grapeseed oil
- ¼ cup of distilled water
- ½ ounce of beeswax
- 8 drops of lavender essential oil
- 8 drops of orange essential oil

1.   Melt the wax with grapeseed oil in a double boil then remove it from the heat and allow it to cool down until it becomes warm to the touch.

2.   Stir in the distilled water with orange floral water then transfer them to a food processor and blend them smoothly.

3.   Add in the essential oils to the lotion mix and blend them for 30 sec.

4.   Transfer the lotion into a mason jar and seal it then use it right away or refrigerate it until ready to use.

5.   You can use this lotion every day especially if you have dry skin, and you can use it on your babies as well.

Nutty Roses Lotion

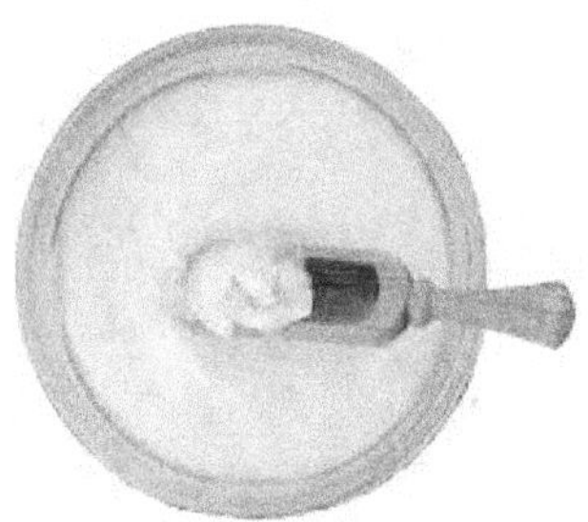

Ingredients:

- 1 cup of raw shea butter
- ½ cup of coconut oil
- ½ cup of sweet almond oil
- 5 drops of carrot seed essential oil
- 5 drops of rosemary essential oil

Directions:

1. Melt the almond oil with butter and coconut oil in a double boiler then stir in the essential oils right away.

2. Chill the lotion in the fridge for 2 h until it hardens then whip it with a hand mixer until it becomes creamy and soft.

3. Transfer the lotion into a mason jar and seal it then use it right away or refrigerate it until ready to use.

4. This lotion will keep your skin moisturized and soft the whole day.

Lavender Roses Lotion

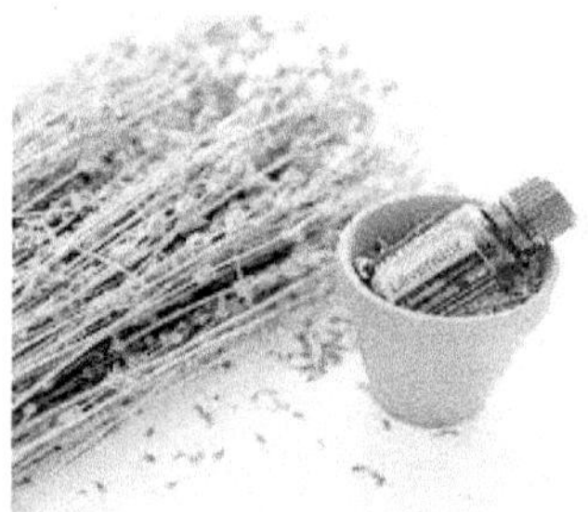

Ingredients:

- 16 ounces of baby lotion
- 8 ounces of Vitamin E cream
- 8 ounces of Vaseline
- 5 drops of rose essential oil
- 5 drops of lavender essential oil

Directions:

1.   Combine all the ingredients in a mixing bowl then whip them until they become creamy.

2.   Transfer the lotion into a mason jar and seal it then use it right away or refrigerate it until ready to use.

3.   This is an incredible moisturizing lotion that will leave your skin smelling heavenly.

Frankincense Vanilla Lotion

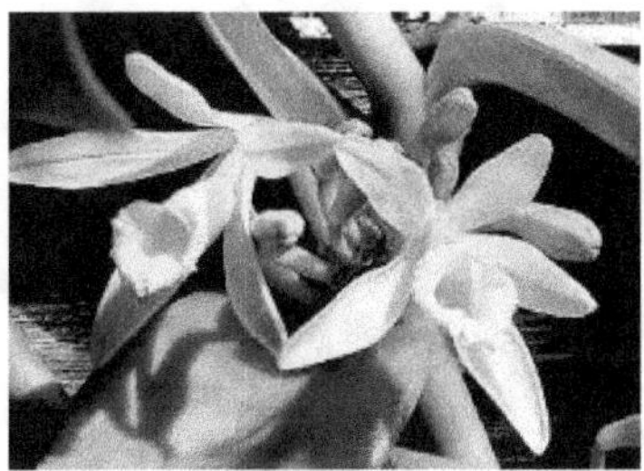

Ingredients:

- 1 cup of olive oil
- ¼ cup of beeswax
- ¼ cup of coconut oil
- 2 tablespoons of cocoa butter
- 1 teaspoon of vitamin E oil
- 5 drops of vanilla essential oil
- 5 drops of frankincense essential oil

Directions:

1.   Stir all the ingredients in the bowl of a double boiler.

2.   Transfer the lotion into a mason jar and seal it then use it right away or refrigerate it until ready to use.

3.   This is an incredible moisturizing lotion that will leave your smelling skin heavenly.

Lavender Lemon Lotion

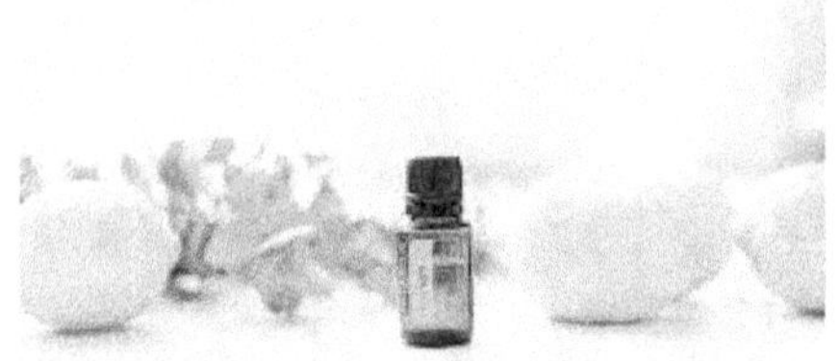

Ingredients:

- 1 cup of aloe vera gel
- ½ cup of sweet almond oil
- ½ cup of beeswax, grated
- 1 teaspoon of vitamin E oil
- 5 drops of lavender essential oil
- 5 drops of lemon essential oil
- 5 drops of Eucalyptus essential oil

Directions:

1.   Whisk the aloe vera gel with vitamin E oil and almond oil in a small bowl then set it aside.

2.   Melt the beeswax in a double boiler then pour it in a food processor and add to it the oils and aloe vera mix.

3.   Cover the processor and blend them smooth then add in the essential oils and blend them again until you get a creamy mix.

4.   This lotion will repair and moisturize your skin, especially in the harsh winter.

Tea Carrot Lotion

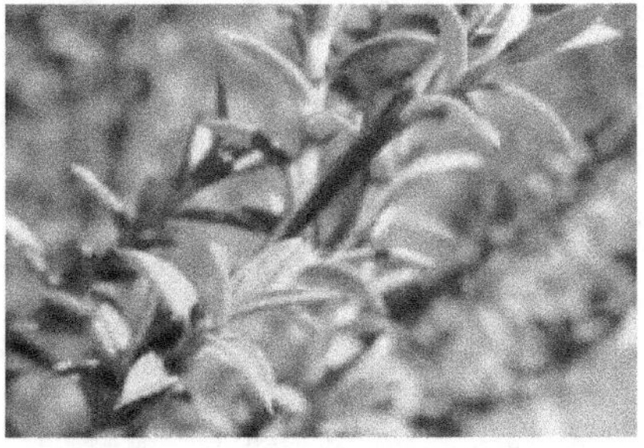

Ingredients:

- 4 ounces of shea butter
- 2 tablespoons of avocado oil
- 10 drops of lavender essential oil
- 5 drops of carrot seed oil
- 5 drops of tea tree essential oil
- 5 drops of rosemary essential oil

Directions:

1.   Place the butter in a saucepan and melt it over low heat then stir into it the avocado oil and remove it from the heat.

2.   Refrigerate the mix for 15 to 20 min until it starts to harden.

3.   Once the time is up, add in the essential oils to the mix and whip them until they become light and creamy.

4.   Transfer the lotion into a mason jar and seal it then use it right away or refrigerate it until ready to use.

5.   This is an incredible moisturizing lotion will nourish your skin and provide with all the vitamins that it needs.

Chamomile Lotion Bar

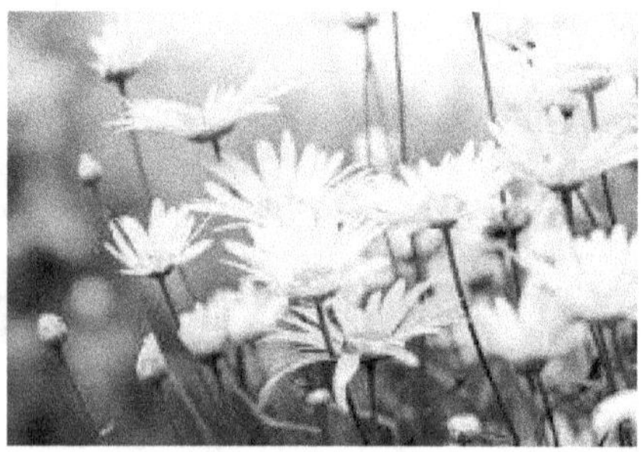

Ingredients:

- 1/8 cup of coconut oil
- 2 1/8 tablespoons of cocoa butter
- 1 1/3 tablespoon of beeswax

- 1 teaspoon of peppermint essential oil
- ½ teaspoon of lavender essential oil
- ¼ teaspoon of rosemary essential oil
- 15 drops of chamomile essential oil

Directions:

1.   Combine the beeswax with cocoa butter and coconut oil in a double boiler and stir them until they completely.

2.   Remove the oils from the heat and stir into it the essential oils.

3.   Transfer the lotion into a mason jar and seal it then use it right away or refrigerate it until ready to use.

4.   This lotion is an amazing moisturizer for your skin; you can use it for your baby as well without worrying about anything.

Chapter 4 – Lotions for Oily Skin

Tropical Creamy Lotion

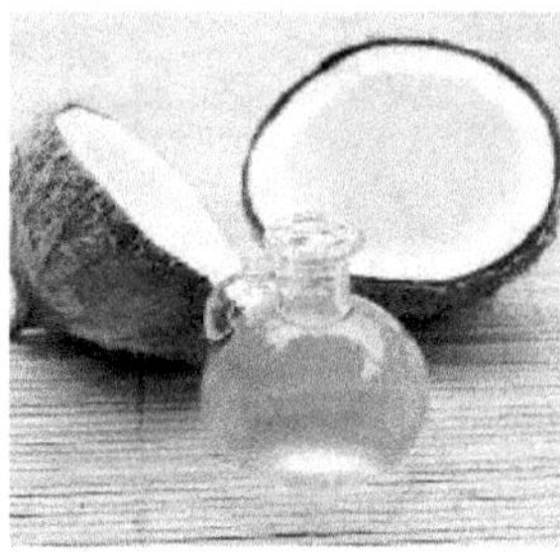

Ingredients:

- ½ cup of coconut oil
- ½ cup of shea butter
- 10 drops of orange essential oil
- 10 drops of lime essential oil
- 5 drops of grapefruit essential oil

Directions:

1.   Melt the shea butter with coconut oil in a double boiler and allow it to cool down for 3 to 5 min.

2.   Add in the essential oils and whip the mix until it becomes creamy then use it after shaving and enjoy.

3.   This lotion will make your skin so soft and fresh not to mention that it will stop the itching feeling that you get after shaving.

Bluish Winter Lotion

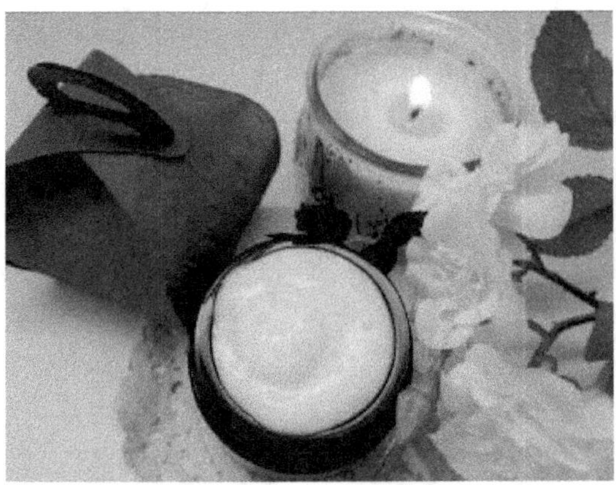

Ingredients:

- 27 ounces of baby lotion
- 8 ounces of coconut oil
- 7 ounces of Aquaphor
- 4 ounces of Fruit of Earth vitamin E cream

Directions:

1. Combine all the ingredients in a large bowl and whip them with a hand mixer until they become creamy.

2. Transfer the mix into a mason jar and refrigerate it then use it whenever you desire.

3. This lotion is perfect for the harsh winter season that leaves your skin chapped and cracked, this lotion will repair your skin and keep it moisturized.

Lavender Facial Lotion

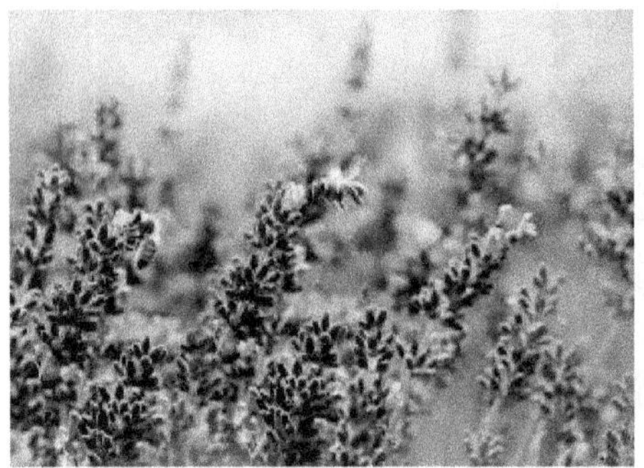

Ingredients:

- 3 ½ tablespoons of shea butter
- 3 tablespoons of ale vera gel
- 2 tablespoons of jojoba oil
- 1 teaspoon of vitamin E oil
- 4 drops of lavender essential oil

Directions:

1. Melt the jojoba oil with butter in a double boiler then stir into them the aloe vera gel and whip them until they become creamy.

2. Add in the rest of the ingredients and whip them for 1 min then transfer the lotion into a mason jar and use it whenever you desire.

3. This lotion is perfect for people that have dry skin; it will leave your skin moisturized and soft.

Creamy Magnesium Lotion

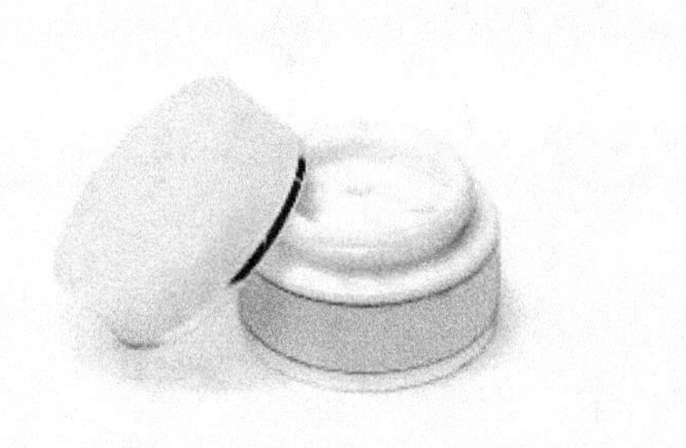

Ingredients:

- ½ cup of magnesium flakes
- ¼ cup of grapes seeds oil
- ¼ cup of coconut oil
- 3 tablespoons of distilled water
- 2 ½ tablespoons of beeswax, grated
- 1 tablespoon of shea butter
- 1 teaspoon of vitamin E oil
- 20 drops of lavender essential oil
- 10 drops of peppermint essential oil

Directions:

1. Bring the water to a boil then remove it from the heat and stir into it the magnesium flakes until it dissolves.

2. Combine the rest of the ingredients in a double boiler and stir them until they completely melt and whip them while adding the magnesium mix until you get a creamy mix.

3.   Transfer the lotion into a mason jar and refrigerate it then use it whenever you desire.

4.   This lotion will nourish your skin and make it healthy as well as relieve your body from all the tension and help you sleep well.

Calming Lavender Lotion

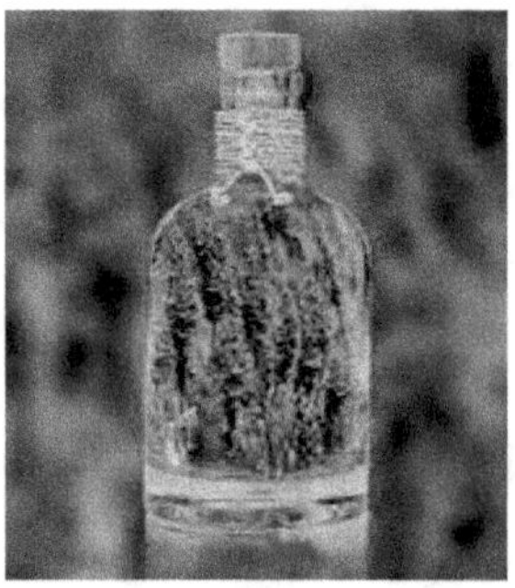

Ingredients:

- ½ cup of organic coconut oil
- 25 drops of lavender essential oil
- 25 drops of Melrose essential oil

Directions:

1.   Melt the coconut oil in a double boiler then stir into it the essential oils and transfer it to a mason jar.

2.   After a long tiring day, this lotion will help you relax and make you feel so good about yourself.

Rosy Shea Lotion

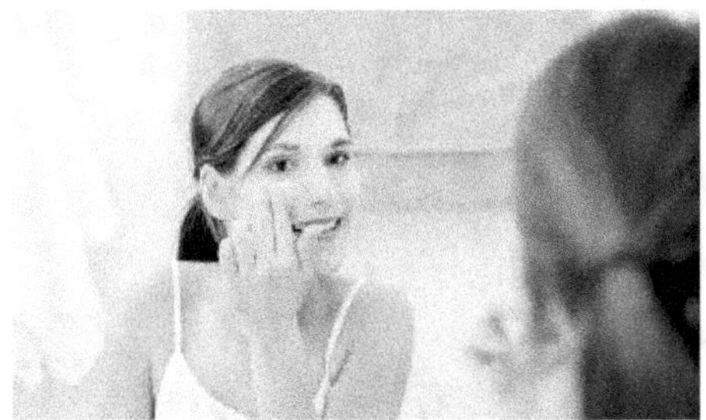

Ingredients:

- ½ cup of shea butter
- 1 tablespoon of almond oil
- 1 tablespoon of jojoba oil
- 10 drops of rosemary essential oil
- 10 drops of lavender essential oil

Directions:

1. Melt the jojoba oil with shea butter and almond oil in a double boiler then refrigerate it for 10 to 15 min.

2. Once the time is up, add in the essential oils and whip the mix with a hand mixer until you get a creamy mix.

3. Transfer your lotion to a mason jar and apply it whenever needed.

4. This lotion will moisturize your skin and prevent it from drying.

Coconut Tea Lotion

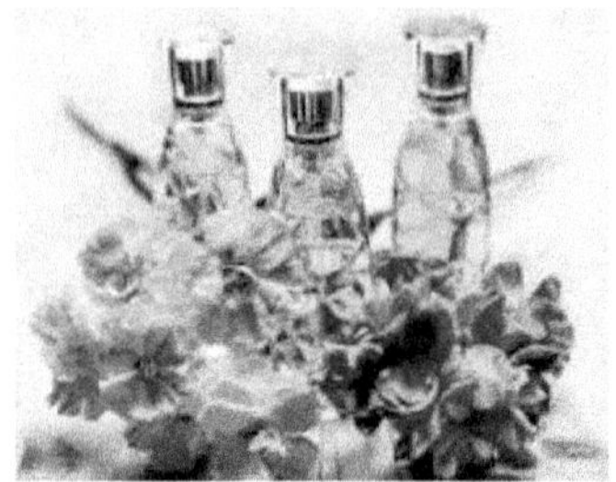

Ingredients:

- ½ cup of shea butter
- 2 tablespoons of avocado oil
- 10 drops of lavender essential oil
- 5 drops of rosemary essential oil
- 3 drops of tea tree essential oil
- 3 drops of carrot seed essential oil

Directions:

1.   Melt the avocado oil with shea butter in a double boiler then refrigerate it for 10 to 15 min.

2.   Once the time is up, add in the essential oils and whip the mix with a hand mixer until you get a creamy mix.

3.   Transfer your lotion to a mason jar and apply it whenever needed.

4.   This lotion will moisturize your skin and keep it looking glowing; you can use it on both your body and face.

Non-greasy Cocoa Lotion

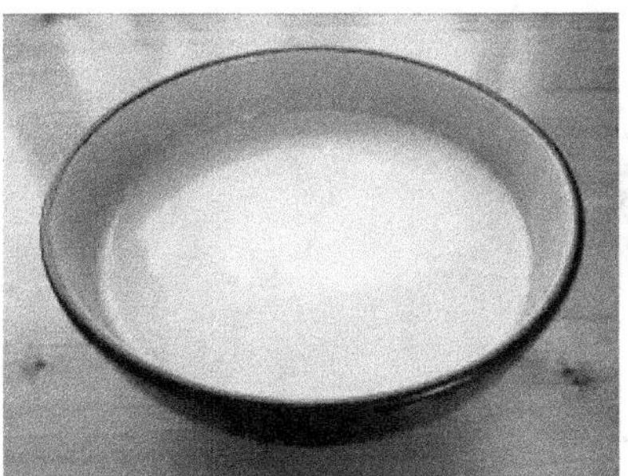

Ingredients:

- ¼ cup of coconut oil
- 1/8 cup of cocoa butter
- 1/8 cup of shea butter
- 1 tablespoon of jojoba oil
- 1 tablespoon of aloe vera juice
- 10 drops of orange essential oil

Directions:

1.   Whisk the essential oil with jojoba oil and aloe vera juice in a small bowl then set it aside.

2.   Combine the rest of the ingredients in a double boiler and melt them completely then stir in the aloe vera mix.

3.   Transfer the lotion into a mason jar and use it whenever you desire.

4.   This lotion will nourish your skin and make it soft.

Creamy Chamomile Lotion

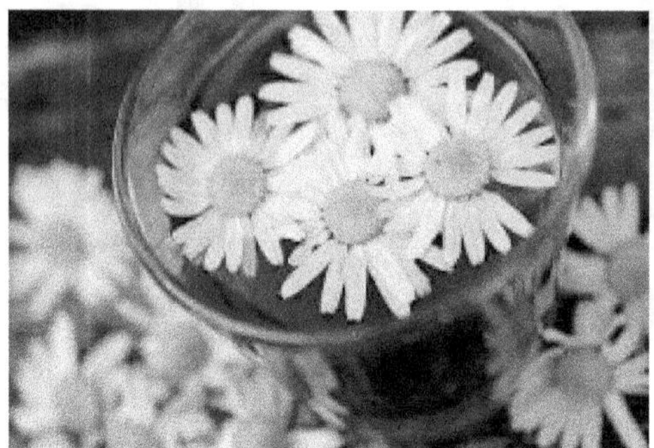

Ingredients:

- 8 ounces of distilled water
- 6 ounces of jojoba oil
- 3 ounces of coconut oil
- 1 ½ ounces of beeswax, grated
- 5 teaspoons of lavender buds
- 5 teaspoons of chamomile flowers

Directions:

1.   Combine the lavender buds with jojoba oil and chamomile flowers in a double boiler then cook them for 2 h on low heat.

2.   Strain the jojoba oil mix through a cheesecloth then combine it with the wax and coconut oil in another double boiler and melt them completely.

3.   Heat the water until it becomes warm to the touch and transfer it into a container then add to it a steady stream of the oils mix while whipping them with an Emerson blender until you get a smooth mix.

4.   Transfer the lotion into a mason jar then use it whenever you want.

5.   This lotion will nourish your skin and soften it as well as calm you and ease all your worries.

Minty Summer Lotion

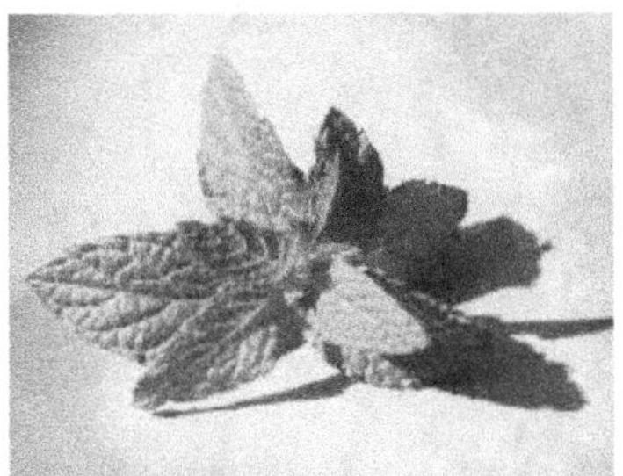

Ingredients:

- ½ cup of aloe vera gel
- ½ cup of coconut oil
- ¼ cup of beeswax, grated
- 1/8 teaspoon of peppermint essential oil

Directions:

1.   Melt the beeswax with coconut oil in a double boiler then whisk in the rest of the ingredients until they become smooth.

2.   Allow the lotion to cool down for 1 h and whisk it again then use it and enjoy.

3.   After a long tiring day in a summer time, this lotion will make you feel cool and keep your skin moisturized.

Eczema Lotion Fighter

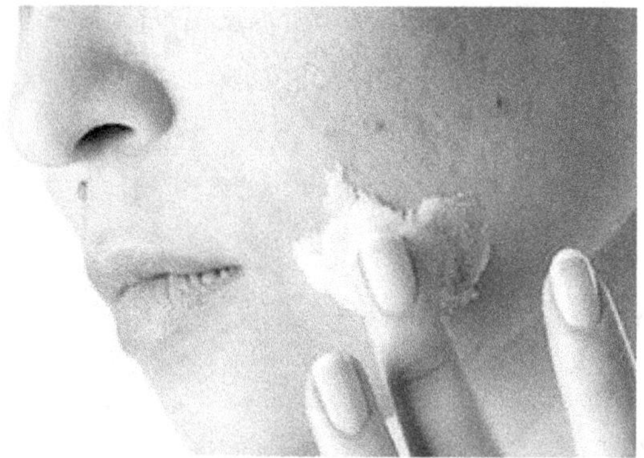

Ingredients:

- ¼ cup of coconut oil
- ¼ cup of shea butter
- 15 drops of lavender essential oil
- 5 drops of tea tree essential oil

Directions:

1.   Melt the coconut oil with shea butter in a double boiler then stir into it the essential oils.

2.   Transfer the lotion into a mason jar and refrigerate it until it hardens then use it whenever you desire and enjoy.

3.   This lotion is high in vitamins so it will contribute to healing your skin from eczema in a fast way.

Creamy Coconut Lotion

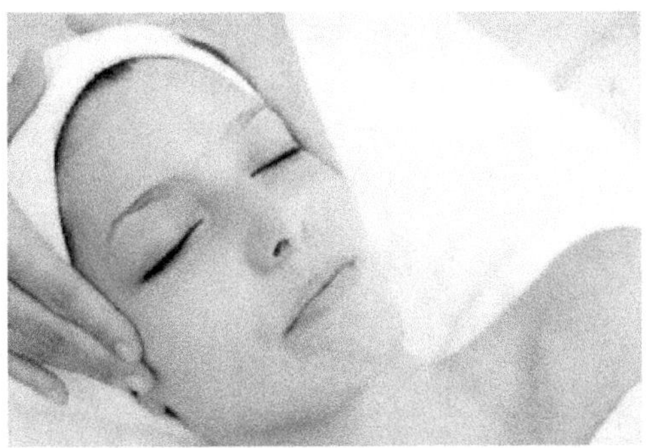

Ingredients:

- ½ cup of beeswax, grated
- ½ cup of fresh aloe vera gel
- ½ cup of distilled water
- ¼ cup of jojoba oil
- ¼ cup of coconut oil
- 1 teaspoon of rosemary extract
- 10 drops of vanilla essential oil
- 5 drops of orange essential oil

Directions:

1. Whisk the water with aloe vera gel and in a bowl and set it aside.

2. Melt the beeswax completely in a double boiler then transfer it with coconut oil, jojoba oil vanilla essential oil, rosemary extract and blend them on the lowest setting.

3. Add in the aloe vera mix in a steady stream to the oils mix while blending them all the time until you get a smooth and creamy mix.

4.   Transfer the lotion into a mason jar and apply it whenever you desire.

5.   This lotion is not greasy at all, apply whenever you are going it or want to go to the beach, it will keep your skin moisturized and protect it from the sun.

Historical Honey Lotion

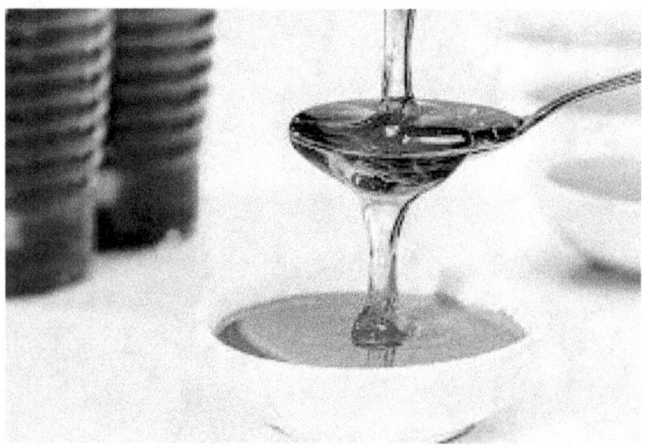

Ingredients:

- 7/8 cups of almond oil
- ½ cup of rose water
- ½ cup tablespoons of beeswax, grated
- 1 tablespoon of raw honey

Directions:

1.   Melt the honey with almond oil and beeswax in a double boiler completely and allow them to cool down for few minutes.

2.   Add the rose water while whisking it all the time then transfer into a mason jar and use it whenever you want.

3.   The lotion will cleanse your face and keep it moisturized.

Wild Rosy Lotion

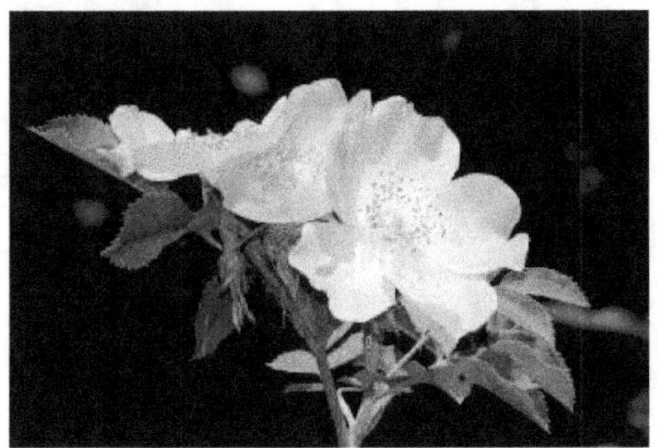

Ingredients:

- 1/3 cup of rosewater
- 1 teaspoon of sunflower oil
- ½ teaspoon of sodium lactate
- ¼ teaspoon of rice bran oil
- ¼ teaspoon of honey

- ¼ teaspoon of liquid Germall plus
- 1/8 teaspoon of cocoa butter
- 20 drops of Vitamin E oil
- 10 drops of geranium essential oil

Directions:

1.   Combine the Germall plus, rose water, sodium lactate and honey in a double boiler and melt them completely.

2.   Heat the rest ingredients in a double boiler until they become warm to the touch then transfer them with the rose water to a mason jar.

3.   Whisk the mix with a coffee whisker until you get a smooth and creamy lotion then refrigerate it and use it whenever you want.

4.   This is an amazing hands lotion that will keep your hands soft and make smell good all day.

Chapter 5 – Sunscreen Lotions

Orange Summer Lotion

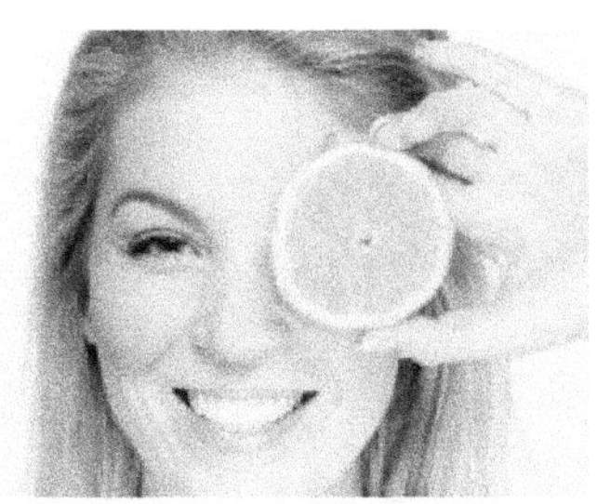

Ingredients:

- ¼ cup of cocoa butter
- 1/8 cup of sweet almond oil
- 1/8 cup of coconut oil
- 25 drops of orange essential oil

Directions:

1. Combine the almond oil with butter and coconut oil in a double boiler and stir them until they completely melt.

2. Remove the oils mix from the heat and stir in the essential oil.

3. Transfer the lotion into a mason jar and allow it to cool down then use it right away or refrigerate it until ready to use.

4. This lotion will moisturize your skin, relieve your stress and make your skin healthier.

Baby Coconut Lotion

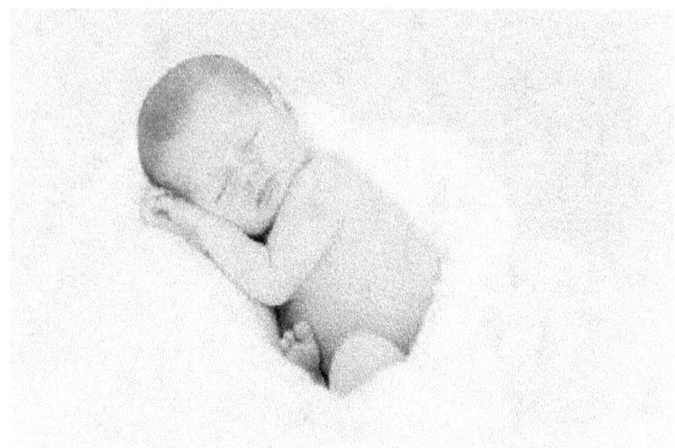

Ingredients:

- 16 ounces of baby lotion
- 8 ounces of vitamin E cream
- 8 ounces of solid coconut oil
- 4 ounces of cocoa butter

Directions:

1.   Combine all the ingredients in a medium bowl and whip them until their soft peaks.

2.   Transfer the mix into a mason jar and seal it then use it right away or refrigerate it until ready to use.

3.   This lotion with make your skin feels amazing.

Aphoristic Lotion

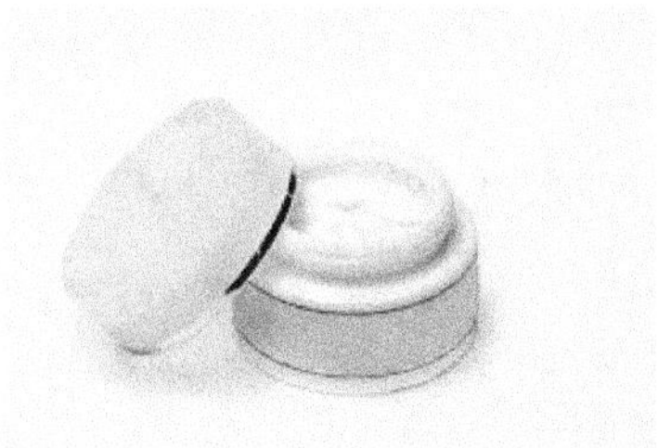

Ingredients:

- ½ cup of grapes seeds oil
- ½ cup of coconut oil
- 1 ounce of beeswax, grated
- ½ ounce of cocoa butter
- ¼ cup of rose hydrosol
- ¼ cup of aloe vera gel
- 1 tablespoon of vitamin E oil
- 1 tablespoon of rosehip seed oil
- 2 teaspoons of Aphrodite aroma oil
- 10 drops of Peru Balsam essential oil

Directions:

1. Combine the grapes seed oil with vitamin E oil, coconut oil, beeswax, cocoa butter with rosehip seed oil in a double boiler then melt them completely.

2. Mix the aloe vera gel with Peru Balsam essential oil in another small bowl then stir them into the oils mix once they cool down and become warm to the touch.

3. Transfer the mix into a food processor and blend them smooth until the lotion becomes thick like a medium thick pudding.

4.   Stir in the Aphrodite aroma oil into the lotion then transfer it to a mason a jar and refrigerate it or use it right away.

5.   If you want a boost of confidence, or you simply want to impress someone, this lotion will leave your skin soft as a baby's and make you smell heavenly.

Jojoba Nut Lotion

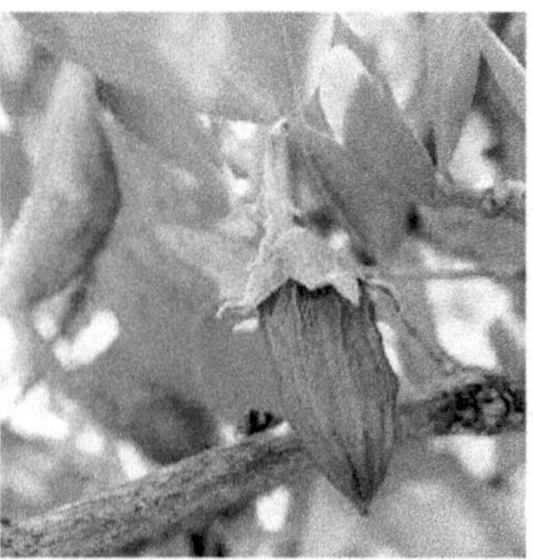

Ingredients:

- ½ cup of jojoba oil
- ½ cup of cocoa butter
- ½ cup of coconut oil

Directions:

1.   Melt the cocoa butter with jojoba oil in a double boiler then stir into them the jojoba oil and remove them from the heat.

2.   Refrigerate the lotion mix for several hours until it starts to firm then whip it with a hand mixer until it becomes creamy.

3.   Transfer the mix into a mason jar and seal it then use it right away or refrigerate it until ready to use.

4.   This lotion will knock off all your store bought lotions and become your favorite because it will moisturize the skin and soften it.

Relaxing Lavender Lotion

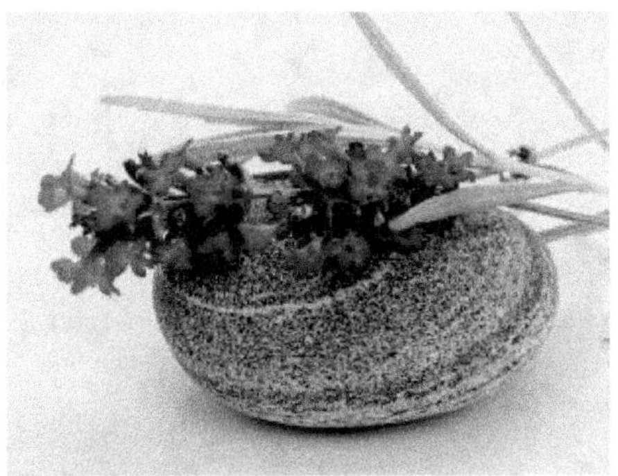

Ingredients:

- 8 ounces of distilled water
- 6 ounces of jojoba oil
- 3 ounces of solid coconut oil
- 1 ½ ounces of beeswax, grated
- 5 drops of chamomile essential oil
- 5 drops of vanilla essential oil

Directions:

1.   Melt the wax with jojoba and coconut oil in a double boiler and stir them until they liquefy.

2.   Heat the water in small saucepan until it becomes warm to the touch then add to it a thin steady stream of oil while whisking all the time with a hand mixer until you get a creamy mix similar to mayonnaise.

3.   Stir in the essential oils and transfer the mix into a mason jar then seal it and use it right away or refrigerate it until ready to use.

4.   After a long tiring day, this lotion removes all the stress from your body as well as helps you relax and sleep better.

Sunny Bee Lotion

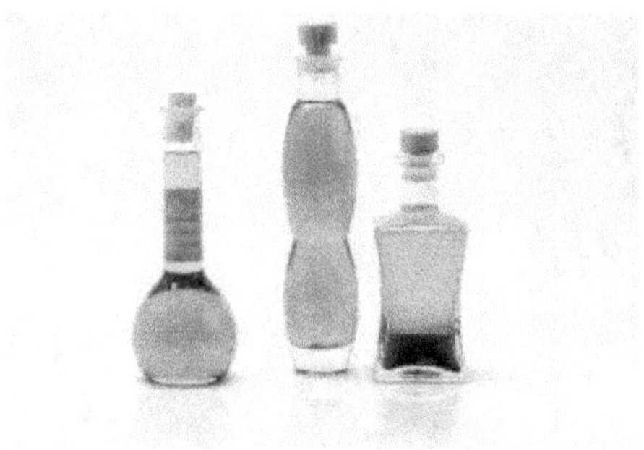

Ingredients:

- ½ cup of sunflower oil
- ¼ cup of boiled water
- 1 tablespoon of beeswax, grated
- 1/8 teaspoon of baking soda

Directions:

1.   Pour the water in a small bowl and dissolve in it the baking soda.

2.   Combine the wax with oil in a double boiler over low heat and stir it until it completely melts.

3.   Heat the soda and water mix until its temperature becomes similar to the oils mix temperature.

4.   Pour the soda and water mix into the oils mix in a steady stream while stirring them all the time.

5.   Allow the lotion to cool down completely while stirring it every once in a while then transfer it to a mason jar and refrigerate it until you want to use it.

6.   This lotion is great for dry skin; it moisturizes it and softens it.

Seductive Vanilla Lotion

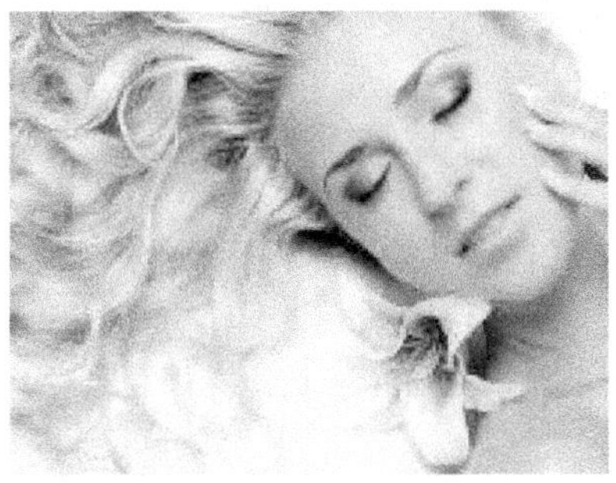

Ingredients:

- ½ cup of olive oil
- ¼ cup of beeswax, grated
- ¼ cup of coconut oil

- 2 tablespoons of cocoa butter
- 1 tablespoon of vitamin E oil
- 2 drops of vanilla extract

Directions:

1.   Combine all the ingredients in a mason jar and put on the lid loosely then place it in a double boiler.

2.   Stir the mix from time to time with a spoon until it completely melts then use it after taking a bath and enjoy.

3.   This lotion will nourish your skin and protect it from eczema; you can use it on your baby as well.

Smooth Clay Lotion

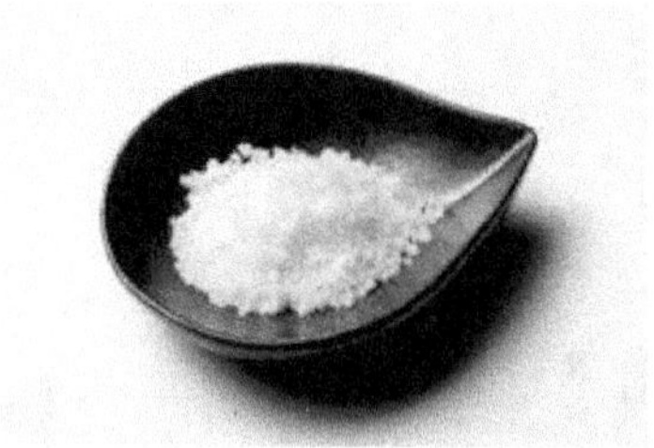

Ingredients:

- 1/8 cup of water
- 1 tablespoon of finely ground sea salt
- 1 tablespoon of baking soda
- 1 tablespoon of bentonite clay
- 1 teaspoon of glycerin

Directions:

1.   Whisk the salt with soda and clay in a small bowl then add in the water followed by the glycerin while whisking all the time until no lumps are found.

2.   Store the lotion in a container and refrigerate it then use it whenever you want and enjoy.

3.   This lotion with smoothen your skin and keeping it from drying.

Sun Blocking lotion

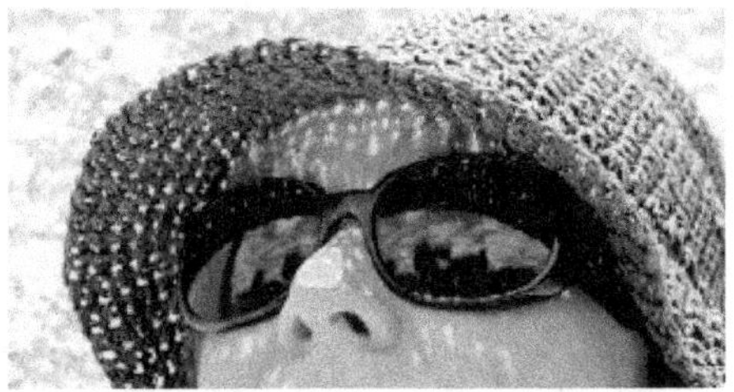

Ingredients:

- 1 ounce of beeswax, grated
- ¼ cup of olive oil
- 2 tablespoons of coconut oil
- 2 teaspoons of shea butter
- 1 teaspoon of vanilla extract

Directions:

1.   Combine the beeswax with coconut oil, butter and olive oil in a double boiler then stir them until they completely melt.

2.   Stir in the vanilla extract into the mix and pour it into a mason jar then use it whenever you want and enjoy.

3.   This lotion will make your skin smooth, protect it from the sun and leave smelling of vanilla.

Natural Sunscreen Lotion

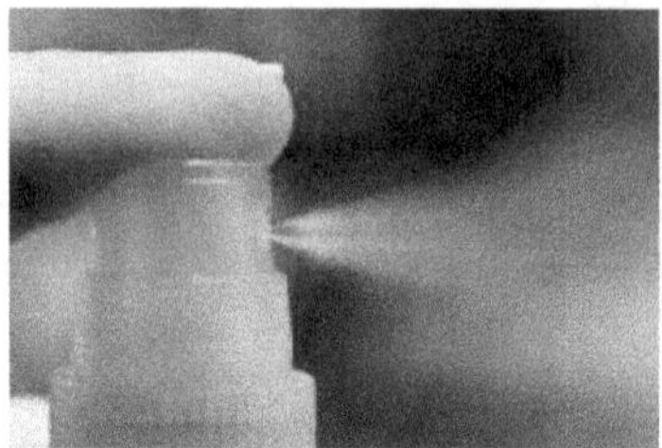

Ingredients:

- 2 ounces of avocado oil
- 2 ounces of beeswax, grated
- 2 ounces of coconut oil
- 1 ounce of shea butter
- 1 ounce of cocoa butter
- 25 drops of lavender essential oil
- 10 drops of carrot seed essential oil
- 10 drops of myrrh essential oil
- 2 drops of sandalwood essential oil

Directions:

1. Combine all the ingredients except for the essential oils in a double boiler and heat them until they melt completely.

2. Stir in the vanilla extract into the mix and pour it into a mason jar then use it whenever you want and enjoy.

3. This lotion will make your skin smooth, nourish it and protect it from the sun.

Aloe Vera Lotion

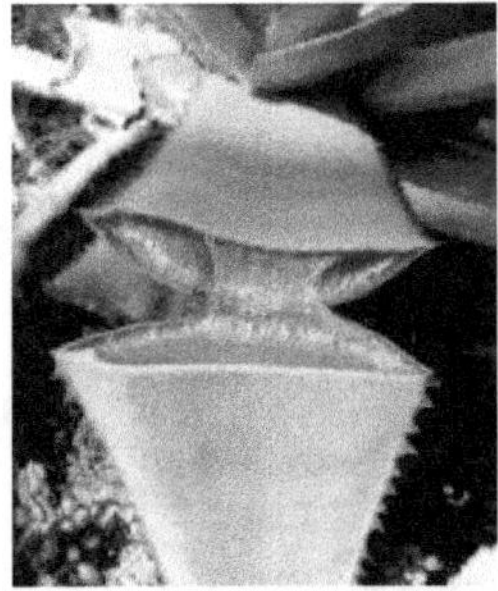

Ingredients:

- 1 cup of pure aloe vera gel
- ½ cup of sweet almond oil
- ½ cup of beeswax, grated
- 1 teaspoon of vitamin E oil
- 15 drops of jasmine essential oil

Directions:

1.   Whisk the essential oil with aloe vera and vitamin E oil in a small bowl and set it aside.

2.   Melt the almond oil with wax in a double boiler then transfer them into a food processor and allow them to cool down for few minutes.

3.   Blend the wax mix on low settings then add in the aloe vera gel gradually while blending them until you are satisfied with the consistency of the lotion.

4.   Transfer the lotion into a mason jar and apply whenever you desire.

5.   This lotion is a great moisturizer for you to use in both summer and winter.

Chapter 6 – Secrets to making natural lotions

If you're like many people who are trending toward more natural health and personal care, learning what's in your lotions and products has become more important than anything else. Here are some secrets to help you make some truly natural lotions and products so you can be sure about what it is you are putting on your skin.

#1: Choosing the Correct Plant

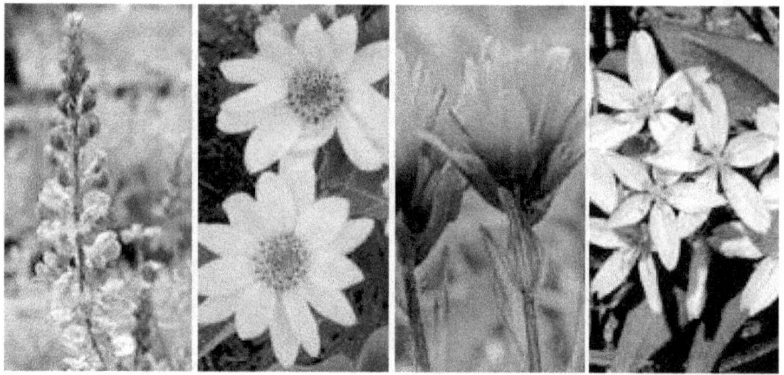

To learn how to make the finest and purest hand-crafted lotions, creams, and skin care products, you first need to know which specific plant ingredients work to balance, repair, and encourage your skin to be its best.

Whether your skin is sensitive, aging, dry, oily, or normal, nature has given us the right plant to correct the problem. Plants all have different properties. Some are astringent or hydrating, others have the ability to absorb moisture or oil, and still others contain properties that mimic human sebum, so choosing the right plant for your skin to include in your homemade lotions is essential.

#2: The Extraction Process

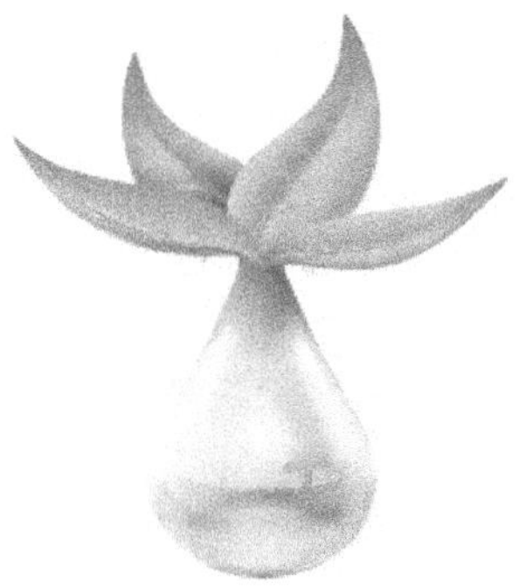

Knowing the properties of plants is the first step to making your own lotions but knowing how to correctly remove those properties from the plant - and which part of the plant to remove them from - is next. Leaves, berries, petals, stems, seeds, and nuts all contribute a specific quality.

Essential oil distillation, infusions, tinctures, decoctions, flower waters, and hydrosols are all used for different reasons in making lotions. They all require differing methods of extraction so the delicate plant properties are not destroyed.

#3: Getting the Desired Texture and Result

Getting oil and water to mix is pure chemistry, but you don't need to be a chemist to keep your lotion ingredients from separating (a process called emulsification). Different consistencies are used for different purposes and the final consistency of your product will be defined as a lotion (hand lotion, body lotion, after shave, cleanser), or a cream (foot cream, eye cream, hand cream, night cream). The result depends on your oil to water ratio and anything less than 20% water will result in an ointment.

There's a lot of information out there about how to take care of your skin and more products than you can ever imagine. Being aware of the characteristics of your skin will go a long way to helping your decide which lotions and products are best for you. Even better, to help you decide which homemade lotion or cream to make for yourself.

Importance of a natural skin lotion

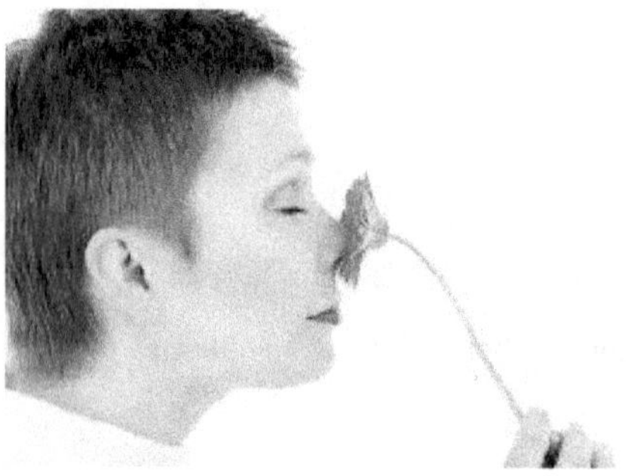

information about an effective and natural skin lotion which can penetrate deep into the skin, nourish it, hydrate it, regenerate it and rejuvenate it. It will also restore the protein balance within the skin. Let us take a look at them one by one.

1. **Nourish and moisturize the skin**- this requirement can be easily met with the natural emollients like Avocado Oil and Maracuja. They have the ability to go deep into the skin and moisturize it inside out. These ingredients have a high nutritional value which is used to nourish the skin and make it healthy from inside.

They also help in regenerating the damaged skin cells, replacing them with the new ones and thus keeping the skin soft, supple and fresh always.

2. **Restore balance among the skin proteins** - this is important to even out the degenerative reactions taking place in the body especially when you are aging.

For example - with age, the production of Collagen and Elastin, which are the proteins responsible for keeping the skin smooth and elastic, goes down and hence you develop wrinkles. If you use a lotion containing Cynergy TK(TM), it can restore the level of Collagen and Elastin and make the skin smooth and wrinkle free again.

Similarly, due to the harmful UV rays from the sun, the production of the skin protein called Melanin goes up and as a result it starts depositing in the skin taking the form of age spots. If you use Extrapone Nutgrass Root, it can inhibit the over production of Melanin and thus prevent age spots from occurring.

So essentially, an ideal skin lotion should focus on - one, providing the skin with necessary nutrients to keep it healthy from within; and two, maintaining the balance of skin proteins so that you stay away from common problems like fine lines, wrinkles, age spots, dry skin etc.

If you want to look out for an effective and perfect skin lotion, make sure to check the list of ingredients that it has. It must have some or all of the powerful natural ingredients discussed above.

Conclusion

Standing in the lotion aisle at the market can be overwhelming. Not only are there hundreds of options to choose from, but if you pick up a bottle and try to decipher what it is made of it's like reading a foreign language. Too many lotions and brands use unrecognizable and unpronounceable ingredients.

Most of these ingredients are chemicals, or synthetic materials that were made in a science lab. While they won't give you any harmful diseases, they can cause skin irritation or allergic reactions. Not only that, but they can even dry your skin out more forcing you to constantly reapply and buy bottle after bottle.

If you have sensitive skin or allergies to fragrances or other allergies, trying to decipher the ingredients on the back of the lotion bottle can make the difference between a good experience and a bad one.

The easiest solution is to bypass this entire process. Make your own organic lotion or body butter and rest easy knowing exactly what is in the lotion you are putting on your skin.

Your skin is the largest organ on the body, it is important to take care of it. It is the first line of defense against the environment, and it keeps everything inside our bodies that we want to stay inside our bodies. Your skin is essential, and caring for it properly should be too.

It may seem daunting to try and make your own lotion, but it is as easy as one, two, and three. It is a less stressful solution by far to make your own lotion or body butter, than it is to go through the intense process of buying one.

Making your own lotion, body butter, or hand cream gives you the ability to meet your own specific and unique skin care needs. No one is exactly the same, and therefore no one's skin is the exact same either. Making your own lotion gives you the chance to create a moisturizer for your skin type with the ingredients that will give your skin the health and protection you want it to.

When you make your own lotion, you have the option of mixing as many or as few ingredients as you want. While the recipes above only require two oils and an optional butter, there's no reason you can't add more.

If you wanted the vitamins of Almond oil, the scent and protection of Apricot oil, and the collagen stimulus of Avocado oil, there's no reason you can't have all three. The key is to make sure that you do the math correctly so that your lotion doesn't turn into too much of a liquid and lose that lotion texture.

Some measurements for you:

Three oils:

- ¼ cup each oil for an equal dose of each.
- ½ cup primary oil, 1/8 cup for second and third oils

Four oils:

- ¼ cup primary oil, 1/8 cup for second, third, and fourth oils.

It is not recommended to add more than four oils, not only because the math gets a little trickier after that, but then the mixture might not mix as well and you risk separation.

Have the peace of mind of knowing exactly what you are putting on your body. Take care of your skin; moisturize it, repair it, heal it, and protect it. Lotion can be so much more than just a skin soother, and when you make your own you can make it that way.

Making your own lotion gives you the chance to fight against your biggest skin concerns, whether those are elasticity and collagen concerns, ultraviolet or UV rays concerns, aging and wrinkle concerns, or severe dry skin like eczema. Making your own lotion means you can make the perfect concoction to address all these issues and give yourself beautiful and healthy skin.

Don't settle for store bought lotions which can dry your skin out more or cause allergic reactions or irritation. Make your own and live life in happy, healthy skin.

Thank you again for downloading this book! I do hope you found these recipes as helpful as I did. You can never go wrong with organic and natural products, and the results will always be surprisingly incredible!!